PMS
WL
18
BEW

Essential Revision Notes in
Clinical Neurology

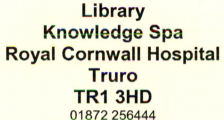
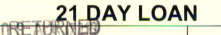

Essential Revision Notes in Clinical Neurology

HANI TS BENAMER
FRCP, PhD
Consultant Neurologist
Honorary Clinical Senior Lecturer
The Royal Wolverhampton Hospitals NHS Trust
University Hospitals NHS Foundation Trust
University of Birmingham

Radcliffe Publishing
London • New York

Radcliffe Publishing Ltd
33–41 Dallington Street
London
EC1V 0BB
United Kingdom

www.radcliffepublishing.com

Electronic catalogue and worldwide online ordering facility.

British Library Cataloguing in Publication Data

A catalogue record for this book is available from the British Library.

ISBN-13: 978 184619 529 7

The paper used for the text pages of this book is FSC® certified. FSC (The Forest Stewardship Council®) is an international network to promote responsible management of the world's forests.

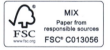

Typeset by Darkriver Design, Auckland, New Zealand
Printed and bound by TJI Digital, Padstow, Cornwall, UK

Contents

About the author

After graduating from Tripoli, Libya, in 1990, Hani came to the United Kingdom in 1991 to further his training in medicine. He obtained the MRCP (Membership of the Royal Colleges of Physicians of the United Kingdom) in 1994 and trained in neurology at the Institute of Neurological Sciences in Glasgow. He obtained a PhD and CCST (Certificate of Completion of Specialist Training) in neurology in 2000, and was appointed a consultant neurologist in Wolverhampton and Birmingham the same year. He has been the lead neurologist at New Cross Hospital in Wolverhampton since 2006.

Hani has an interest in medical education, and obtained a post-graduate certificate in the field from Keele University, Staffordshire, in 2007. He has published more than 30 papers, and is currently one of the editors of the *Libyan Journal of Medicine*. He was also an examiner for the MRCP (UK) Diploma from 2005 to 2009.

Preface

Neurological disorders account for 10% of consultations in primary care and 20% of acute hospital admissions. However, there is good evidence that 'neurophobia' is common among medical students leading to the well-established reputation of neurology being a difficult subject. One of the reasons for the neurophobia is the ease with which medical students can get lost in unnecessary details, not concentrating on the most common and basic neurological problems – that is, getting bogged down in detail! This book was put together to help overcome this problem.

Essential Revision Notes in Clinical Neurology is limited to the fundamental knowledge of common and important neurological disorders, hence omitting the unnecessary details or subjects. The book is divided into four sections: Part I introduces the reader to clinical neurology by covering the basic aspects of a neurological consultation, including history and examination; Part II covers neurological signs related to cranial nerves, motor and sensory system and peripheral nerve lesions; Part III covers the major and common neurological problems and diseases (the big five – headache, epilepsy, stroke, Parkinson's disease and multiple sclerosis); Part IV covers other main neurological problems and diseases.

Deliberately, this book contains no diagrams or photos! There is a plethora of excellent neurology textbooks on the market that contain all the classic neurological diagrams such as different types of visual field defects. In the era of the internet, looking at clinical signs such as cranial nerve palsy in printed format is probably less useful than looking at live records on YouTube.

This book is targeted towards medical students and can be used for revision. However, it could also be useful as a first read if the learner has some background knowledge in neurology through attending neurology lectures, bedside teaching and outpatient clinics during the internal medicine and neurology attachments.

I hope the book lives up to its aim of detailing basic principles while omitting unnecessary details and, therefore, I also hope it proves to be good company for medical students, as well as helping to demystify neurology.

Hani TS Benamer
June 2011

Acknowledgements

I would like to thank Dr John Winer, who kindly provided me with constructive comments on the manuscript.

Abbreviations

ABC	Airway, Breathing, Circulation
AD	Alzheimer's disease
ADEM	acute disseminated encephalomyelitis
AED	antiepileptic drug
APD	afferent pupillary defect
CIDP	chronic inflammatory demyelinating polyradiculoneuropathy
CMT	Charcot–Marie–Tooth disease
CNS	central nervous system
COMT	catechol-O-methyl transferase
CSF	cerebrospinal fluid
CT	computerised tomography
CTA	computerised tomographic angiography
CTV	computerised tomographic venogram
CVST	cerebrovenous sinus thrombosis
ECG	electrocardiogram
EEG	electroencephalogram
EMG	electromyography
ENT	ear, nose and throat
ESR	erythrocyte sedimentation rate
ET	essential tremor
GBS	Guillain–Barré syndrome

GCS	Glasgow Coma Scale
HD	Huntington's disease
IV	intravenous
LMN	lower motor neurone
LP	lumbar puncture
MAOB	monoamine oxidase B
MG	myasthenia gravis
MND	motor neurone disease
MRA	magnetic resonance angiography
MRI	magnetic resonance imaging
MRV	magnetic resonance venogram
MS	multiple sclerosis
NCS	nerve conduction study
NMO	neuromyelitis optica
PCR	polymerase chain reaction
PD	Parkinson's disease
PET	positron emission tomography
PNS	peripheral nervous system
RAPD	relative afferent pupillary defect
SPECT	single-photon emission computerised tomography
SUDEP	sudden unexpected death in epilepsy
TBM	tuberculous meningitis
TIA	transient ischaemic attack
UMN	upper motor neurone

To the two stars of my life,
my sons: Sherief and Aly

PART I

Introduction to clinical neurology

CHAPTER 1

The neurological consultation

The neurological consultation usually has the following stages.

➤ *Greeting*: welcome the patient and introduce yourself.

➤ *History*:

> ➣ Opening – start by asking 'Tell me about your symptoms' rather than 'Your doctor referred you because of . . . (e.g. headache), tell me about it'. The patient's agenda may differ markedly from the referring doctor's.

> ➣ Exploring – ask direct questions to explore the possible cause of the patient's symptoms: 'How often do you have headaches?'

> ➣ Generating a diagnosis or differential diagnosis – by the end of the history taking, you should have a clear idea of the possible explanation(s) for the patient's symptoms.

➤ *Examination*: no neurologist does a full and detailed neurological examination on any one patient to begin with. The examination is usually *focused* and guided by diagnosis or differential diagnosis generated from the history. There is no point in doing a detailed sensory examination on a patient with a headache! Contrary to popular belief, neurological examination rarely provides a diagnosis; rather, it usually supports the history findings.

➤ *Conclusions*: formulate a plan that may include investigations. Explain the plan to the patient. Ask the patient if they would like to ask any questions.

CHAPTER 2

History

➤ The history taking in neurology is similar to any other subject. However, because some of the major neurology disorders, such as epilepsy, are diagnosed mainly on the history, history taking carries greater importance in neurology than in some other subjects.

➤ It is important to obtain a precise understanding of the patient's symptoms. For example, dizziness could mean lightheadedness, vertigo or even episodes of loss of consciousness.

➤ Details of the onset of the symptoms could help in determining the pathological processes:
  ➤ sudden onset – vascular
  ➤ gradual onset – degenerative
  ➤ paroxysmal – epilepsy or migraine.

➤ Other components of the history could also be helpful in making the diagnosis:
  ➤ family history in genetic disorders
  ➤ excess alcohol intake in peripheral neuropathy
  ➤ drug history such as antipsychotic agents in (drug-induced) Parkinsonism.

➤ Handedness is important, especially in patients with speech symptoms (*see* Chapter 5).

CHAPTER 3

Basic neuroanatomy

➤ Although some basic neuroanatomy is needed to practise clinical neurology, comprehensive knowledge in neuroanatomy is not usually required.

➤ There are 12 cranial nerves:
  - ➤ olfactory (1st) nerve
  - ➤ optic (2nd) nerve
  - ➤ oculomotor (3rd) nerve
  - ➤ trochlear (4th) nerve
  - ➤ trigeminal (5th) nerve
  - ➤ abducent (6th) nerve
  - ➤ facial (7th) nerve
  - ➤ vestibulocochlear (8th) nerve
  - ➤ glossopharyngeal (9th) nerve
  - ➤ vagus (10th) nerve
  - ➤ accessory (11th) nerve
  - ➤ hypoglossal (12th) nerve.

➤ The nervous system is divided into the central nervous system (CNS) and the peripheral nervous system (PNS).

➤ CNS lesions usually cause upper motor neurone (UMN) signs:
  - ➤ increased tone (spasticity)
  - ➤ weakness with no wasting

➤ brisk reflexes and clonus
➤ upgoing plantars.
➤ PNS lesions usually cause lower motor neurone (LMN) signs:
  ➤ reduced tone (spasticity)
  ➤ weakness, wasting and fasciculation
  ➤ reduced or absent reflexes
  ➤ downgoing (normal) plantars.
➤ Anatomically the CNS consists of:
  ➤ brain – including cerebral hemispheres (frontal, parietal, temporal and occipital lobes), brainstem (midbrain, pons and medulla), basal ganglia and cerebellum
  ➤ spinal cord – has three segments (cervical, thoracic and lumbar) and usually ends at the level of L1 vertebra.
➤ Anatomically the PNS consists of:
  ➤ nerve roots including the cauda equina (the nerve roots from the lower end of the spinal cord)
  ➤ plexus (brachial and lumbosacral)
  ➤ nerves
  ➤ neuromuscular junction
  ➤ muscles.
➤ The function of different lobes of the brain is as follows:
  ➤ Frontal – contains the precentral gyrus, which controls the motor function on the opposite side of the body (motor cortex). Also, the dominant hemisphere contains the Broca's area (inferior frontal gyrus), which controls the speech output. The frontal lobe controls the emotions.
  ➤ Parietal – contain the postcentral gyrus, which controls the sensory function on the opposite side of the body (sensory cortex).
  ➤ Temporal – controls the memory. Also, the dominant hemisphere contains the Wernicke's area (superior temporal gyrus), which controls the comprehension of speech.
  ➤ Occipital – controls the vision.
➤ The following are important tracts:
  ➤ Corticospinal (motor pathway) tract – starts at the motor cortex (precentral gyrus), descends through anterior part of

the internal capsule, crosses to the other side in the medulla, travels the spinal cord in the lateral column and terminates in the ventral horn motor neurons.

➤ Spinothalamic (pain and temperature) tract – pain and temperature fibres enter the spinal cord at the dorsal horn, cross to the opposite side and ascend through lateral column to the thalamus, then project through the posterior part of the internal capsule to the sensory cortex (postcentral gyrus).

➤ Dorsal column (position and vibration) – position and vibration sense fibres enter the spinal cord at the dorsal horn, ascend through the posterior (dorsal) column to the medulla, then cross to the other side to project through the posterior part of the internal capsule to the sensory cortex (postcentral gyrus).

➤ It is important to remember that the body is represented upside down in both the sensory and the motor cortex. Both the sensory and the motor cortex functions are contralateral (controlling opposite sides of the body).

CHAPTER 4

Mental state examination

➤ The mini-mental state examination is widely used as a screening tool for mental state. It includes the following components.

➤ *Orientation = 10*
  - Can you tell me today's date/month/year? = 3
  - Which day of the week is it today? = 1
  - Can you tell me which season it is? = 1
  - What city/town are we in? = 1
  - What is the county/country? = 2
  - What building are we in and on what floor? = 2

➤ *Registration = 3*
  - Can you repeat the following (name to the patient three objectives such as 'ball, car, man')? = 3 (one point for each word).

➤ *Attention and calculation = 5*
  - From 100 keep subtracting 7. Give one point for each correct answer. Stop after 5 answers (93/86/79/72/65).
  - Alternatively, ask the patient to spell 'WORLD' backwards and give a point for each correct letter.

➤ *Recall = 3*
  - What are the three words I asked you to say earlier ('ball, car, man')? = 3 (one point for each word).

➢ *Language, naming and repeating = 3*
- Name these objects (show, for example, a watch and pencil). Give one point for each correct answer.
- Repeat the following: 'no ifs, ands or buts'.

➢ *Reading = 2*
- Write the following instruction on a card 'close your eyes'. Ask the patient to read the sentence and do what it says.

➢ *Three-stage command = 3*
- Present the patient with a piece of paper and ask them to take the paper in their left hand, fold it in half and put it on the floor. Give one point for each correct action.

➢ *Construction = 1*
- Draw two intersected hexagons and ask the patient to copy it.

➤ Points total 30. A score below 24 is considered to be abnormal.

CHAPTER 5

Examination of the speech

- ➤ The cortical area of speech is in the dominant hemisphere (left hemisphere in right-handed people and 60%–70% of left-handed people).
- ➤ The speech has four components: comprehension of the language, production of language, articulation of the speech and phonation (sound and volume).
- ➤ Dysphasia is the impairment of comprehension or production of language, dysarthria is the impairment of articulation, and dysphonia is the impairment of phonation.
- ➤ The anatomy of speech includes the following:
    - ➢ superior temporal gyrus (Wernicke's area)
    - ➢ inferior frontal gyrus (Broca's area)
    - ➢ arcuate fasciculus (perisylvian region), which connect the superior temporal gyrus with the inferior frontal gyrus
    - ➢ motor input from corticobulbar pathway, cerebellum and basal ganglia
    - ➢ cranial nerve input such as 10th nerve (supplies the larynx), 12th nerve (supplies the tongue).
- ➤ The two most important aspects in examination of speech are comprehension (understanding) and fluency (spontaneous speech). These should be examined together by:

➢ *Asking questions*
- What is your address?
- What do you do for a living?
- What did you have for breakfast today?
- Ask the patient to describe their job or what they have eaten in some detail to help assess the speech.

➢ *Giving commands*
- Start with simple commands and increase the complexity as appropriate.
- Close your eyes.
- Show me your right hand.
- Close your right eye and touch your left ear with your right hand.

➢ *Assessing repetition*
- Ask the patient to repeat a simple word such as pen or watch.
- Try a full sentence: 'It is very cold today'.
- Try a complicated phrase: 'no ifs, ands or buts'.

➤ Receptive (sensory, fluent, Wernicke's, posterior) aphasia (dysphasia) – patient's comprehension is impaired. The speech is very fluent but does not make any sense (unintelligible), hence receptive aphasia; if it is an isolated finding, patient could be mislabelled as confused. Repetition is impaired. Receptive aphasia is due to a lesion in the superior temporal gyrus in the dominant (left) hemisphere.

➤ Expressive (motor, non-fluent, Broca's, anterior) aphasia (dysphasia) – patient's comprehension is preserved but the speech is not fluent. Repetition is impaired. Expressive aphasia is due to a lesion in the inferior frontal gyrus in the dominant (left) hemisphere.

➤ A lot of patients usually have a combination of both types of aphasia (global aphasia).

➤ Naming is impaired in all forms of aphasia; therefore, it is not usually of any localisation value.

➤ Isolated impairment in repetition is called conductive aphasia and is usually due to a lesion in the arcuate fasciculus.
➤ Causes of aphasia are usually stroke and brain tumours.

CHAPTER 6

Cranial nerves examination

➤ Traditionally the examination of the cranial nerves is conducted according to their numerical order. However, it is a lot easier and more practical if the cranial nerves are examined together as suggested here (the olfactory (1st) nerve is ignored!).

INSPECTION

➤ Reduced forehead wrinkles (7th).
➤ Ptosis (3rd).
➤ Wasting of the temporalis muscles (5th).
➤ Absence of the nasolabial folds (7th).

ASK THE PATIENT TO . . .

➤ Raise the eyebrows (7th).
➤ Shut the eyes tightly. You should try to force them open (7th).
➤ Blow out the cheeks (7th).
➤ Show the teeth or smile (7th).

EXAMINE THE EYES

➤ Be sure that the patient can see by checking their visual acuity using a (pocket) Snellen chart, with glasses. If a Snellen chart is not available, a newspaper or something similar could be used (2nd).

➤ Look at the size of the pupils and their reaction to light, direct and indirect responses (2nd/3rd).
➤ Check the eye movements and ask if there is double vision (3rd, 4th, 6th).
➤ Examine the fundi, mainly looking at the optic discs (2nd).

EXAMINE THE FACE
➤ Test pinprick sensation in the upper, middle and lower parts of the face (the three divisions of the 5th).
➤ Palpate the masseter and temporalis muscles by asking the patient to clench the teeth (5th).

EXAMINE THE MOUTH
➤ Open the jaw against your hand (5th).
➤ Inspect the tongue inside the floor of the mouth (12th).
➤ Ask the patient to protrude the tongue (12th).
➤ Ask the patient to move the tongue from side to side and look for any slowness (12th).
➤ Ask the patient to say 'Ah' and assess the movement of the soft palate and the uvula (10th).

EXAMINE THE NECK AND SHOULDERS
➤ Ask the patient to twist the head to one side against your hand. Palpate the opposite sternomastoid (11th).
➤ Ask the patient to shrug the shoulders against resistance (11th).

OTHERS (OCCASIONALLY NEEDED IN CLINICAL PRACTICE)
➤ Examine the visual field by confrontation. Use a white hatpin (in clinical practice the majority of neurologists use their finger!), sit at the same level as the patient, about one metre away, compare your field to the patient and test the four quadrants. A red pin is used to test for central scotoma.
➤ Test the reaction of the pupils to convergence by asking the patient to look straight ahead and then at the tip of their nose.
➤ If you find evidence of 5th nerve impairment check the corneal reflex. Remember to stimulate the cornea, not the sclera.

➤ If patient has hearing problems, test for evidence of sensorineural deafness (8th):

> *Rinne's test* – strike a 256 or 512 Hz tuning fork and hold in front of the external auditory meatus and then against the mastoid. In the affected ear, air conduction < bone conduction in conductive deafness and air conduction > bone conduction in sensorineural deafness.

> *Weber's test* – strike a 256 or 512 Hz tuning fork and place in the middle of the forehead. The sound will be louder in the affected ear in conductive deafness, and in the normal ear in sensorineural deafness.

CHAPTER 7

Upper limbs examination

INSPECTION

➤ Ask the patient to place their upper limbs outstretched in front of them with their eyes closed and palms facing upwards (pronator test). This will give you a quick idea about any problems with power (drifting down), position sense (fingers move up and down – pseudoathetosis) or cerebellar disease (arms move up).
➤ Muscle wasting.
➤ Muscle fasciculation.
➤ Scars could be relevant (burn marks may suggest syringomyelia).
➤ Check the patient's back for spinal scars or scapular winging.

TONE

➤ Ensure the patient is not in pain.
➤ Ensure the patient is relaxed.
➤ Move each upper limb passively. Feel the tone mainly at the elbow and the wrist by flexing and extending the joints.
➤ Feel for the 'supinator catch' at the wrist by supinating and pronating the forearm.

POWER

➤ Check shoulder abduction (deltoid, C5) by asking the patient to form a wing and resist you from pushing down on their shoulders.

➤ Check the elbow flexion (biceps, C5/6) by asking the patient to pull the supinated forearm against your hand. Then ask the patient to pull the forearm (midway between pronation and supination) against your hand (brachioradialis, C5/6).

➤ Check the elbow extension (triceps, C7) by asking the patient to push the forearm against your hand.

➤ Check finger extension (extensor digitorum, C7) by asking the patient to keep the fingers straight and stop you from pressing them down.

➤ Check the first dorsal interosseous muscle (T1) by asking the patient to push the index finger against your finger.

➤ Check the abductor pollicis brevis (T1) by asking the patient to move the thumb towards the ceiling against your thumb.

REFLEXES

➤ Use the full length of the tendon hammer and let it swing fully.

➤ Check biceps (C5), supinator (C6) and triceps (C7) reflexes. Look for muscle contraction, not only the jerky movement.

COORDINATION

➤ Demonstrate to the patient how to do the finger-to-nose test by taking the patient's finger, pointing to the nose and then to your finger tip.

➤ Now ask the patient to do it.

CHAPTER 8

Lower limbs examination

INSPECTION

➤ Muscle wasting.
➤ Muscle fasciculation.
➤ Any deformities such as pes cavus or asymmetry of the leg length (one leg shorter than the other).
➤ Any scars, usually not relevant!
➤ Check the patient's back for spinal scars.

TONE

➤ Ensure the patient is not in pain.
➤ Feel the tone at the knee by passively and rapidly flexing and extending the knee.
➤ Check the tone at the ankle by flexing and dorsiflexing the foot.
➤ Check the ankle clonus at the same time by holding the knee in a semiflexed position and pushing the foot up suddenly with moderate force.

POWER

➤ Check the hip flexion (L1/2) by asking the patient to push the thigh against your hand with the knee flexed at 90 degrees.
➤ Check knee flexion (L5/S1) by asking the patient to bend the

knee against your hand. Ask then for the knee to be pushed out against your hand to test knee extension (L3/4).

➤ Check the ankle dorsiflexion (L4/5) by asking the patient to push the foot up against your hand. Also check the ankle plantar flexion (S1) by asking the patient to push the foot down against your hand.

REFLEXES

➤ Use the full length of the tendon hammer and let it swing fully.
➤ Check knee (L3/4) and ankle (S1) reflexes. Look for the muscle contraction, not only the jerky movement.
➤ Test the plantar response. Use the orange stick, not the sharp end of the tendon hammer. Start with the lateral side of the foot and move towards the base of the big toe.

COORDINATION

➤ Demonstrate to the patient how to do the heel-to-shin test by taking the heel of the patient, putting it just below the knee and running it down the shin and taking it up again below the knee.
➤ Now ask the patient to do it.

CHAPTER 9

Points to remember

➤ Take time to explain to the patient each step of the examination (e.g. the heel-to-shin test). This will save time and ensure correct technique.
➤ It is important to use the Medical Research Council scale when describing muscle weakness:
  ➢ grade 0 – no *visible* contraction
  ➢ grade 1 – flicker of contraction
  ➢ grade 2 – movement with gravity
  ➢ grade 3 – movement against gravity
  ➢ grade 4 – movement against partial resistance
  ➢ grade 5 – normal power.
➤ Grade the power according to the maximum power achieved.
➤ When examining muscle power, test each side and then compare.
➤ There is no need to do hip extension, adduction or abduction, foot inversion or eversion and extension of the big toe, unless clinically indicated. Examination of muscles such as serratus anterior, rhomboids, supraspinatus and infraspinatus is rarely needed in routine neurological examination.
➤ When reflexes are absent, reinforce by asking the patient to clench their teeth or to hold the fingers of both hands together and pull the hands against each other.

➤ Grade the reflexes as absent, normal or brisk.
➤ Remember that asymmetry of reflexes is usually significant.
➤ Ankle reflex could be elicited by the plantar strike technique. Place your fingers on the sole of the patient's foot, which should be in a passive dorsiflexed position, and strike your fingers.

CHAPTER 10

Sensory examination

➤ Remember that the main purposes of the sensory examination
 are:
  ➤ to identify any sensory level
  ➤ to identify any evidence of glove and stocking distribution
  ➤ to determine any dermatomal impairments.
➤ Always teach the patient first by starting at the sternum or the
 forehead. The patient needs to recognise normal sensation!
➤ Test the pain sensation by using a disposable neurological
 pin.
➤ When examining upper limbs, start at the hand and work up;
 when examining lower limbs, start at the feet and work up.
➤ Testing random points covering the outer and inner aspects of
 the hands, forearms and the arms should cover all dermatomes
 of the upper limbs.
➤ Testing random points covering the outer and inner aspects of
 the feet, calves and the thighs should cover all dermatomes of
 the lower limbs.
➤ Test for joint position sense. Hold the distal interphalangeal
 joint of the middle finger between your two fingers from the
 sides and move it up and down. Make only a small movement
 (2–3 mm) and avoid putting the joint in extreme positions. First
 show the patient what you are going to do and then do it with

patient's eyes closed. Do the same for the lower limbs by holding the big toe at the sides and moving it up and down.

➤ Test for vibration sense. Start with the wrist and if abnormal move to the elbow and shoulder in the upper limbs. Alternatively, start with the ankle (medial malleolus) and if abnormal move to the knee and iliac crest in the lower limbs.

➤ When you examine pinprick sensation, ask the patient, 'Does the pin feel sharp as it did on your chest or forehead?' *Not* 'Do you feel it?' as the answer will always be yes!

➤ There is no need to ask the patient to close their eyes during the pinprick examination as it serves no purpose. However, some general physicians still insist on teaching this to students!

➤ If there is dermatomal impairment of pinprick, please map the abnormality (e.g. L5/S1).

➤ Test the vibration sense with a 128 Hz tuning fork.

➤ Light touch examination does not usually add anything.

CHAPTER 11

Gait examination

➤ Look very carefully at the gait base (wide or narrow?), the steps, the arms (do they swing?), posture (stooped?) and the ability to turn.
➤ Ask the patient to do the tandem walk (heel-to-toe). Demonstrate this to the patient first.
➤ If you think the patient is ataxic, perform Romberg's test. Ask the patient to stand with feet together, arms by the sides, and then ask the patient to close their eyes. Romberg's sign tends to be overrated. All patients with ataxia tend to get worse when they close their eyes. Romberg's sign should only be considered positive if there is a significant degree of worsening of the ataxia after closing the eyes, which indicates sensory ataxia.
➤ Always stand close to the patient when examining tandem gait or performing Romberg's test. You don't want the patient to fall during the examination.
➤ The following are the classic gait abnormalities:
  ➢ *Hemiplegic gait* – the lower limb moves in a semicircle, the toe scraping the floor with each step, and the arm is held in a flexed position close to the chest.
  ➢ *Spastic gait* – a stiff, scissor gait with the legs crossing in front of each other while walking.
  ➢ *Ataxic gait* – patient's gait is wide-based 'drunken gait' with

difficulty performing heel-to-toe test. Patients with sensory ataxia usually have severe impairment of joint position and vibration. Patients usually stamp their feet on the floor when walking. Sensory ataxia is usually due to subacute combined degeneration of the cord (vitamin B_{12} deficiency).

➤ *Parkinsonian gait* – patient walks with small steps and shuffles. Patient stoops with lack of arm swing and the arms are held in flexed positions.

➤ *Steppage gait* – patient lifts the foot high during walking to avoid scraping the toes and foot slapping. This is due to foot drop.

➤ *Waddling gait* – There is lumbar lordosis and the patient's legs are wide apart. The trunk moves from side to side with the pelvis dropping. This is usually due to hereditary muscular dystrophies.

➤ *Gait apraxia, marche à petits pas and lower-body Parkinsonism* – different terms describing patients with difficulty in starting to walk with small, shuffling steps. This is an indication of diffuse cerebrovascular ischaemic disease (small-vessel disease).

CHAPTER 12

Neurological investigations

➤ Neurologists use a whole range of investigations. This chapter provides a brief outline only, as detailed descriptions of these investigations are beyond the scope of this book.

NEURORADIOLOGY

➤ Computerised tomography (CT) scan: easily available and commonly used in emergencies. However, it exposes the patient to a relatively large dose of X-ray. CT is useful in detecting an intracranial bleed, but not helpful in detecting demyelinating plaques or spinal cord pathology. Computerised tomographic angiography (CTA) and computerised tomographic venogram (CTV) are useful in demonstrating abnormalities in intracranial blood vessels such as arterial aneurysm or venous thrombosis.

➤ Magnetic resonance imaging (MRI) scan: does not involve doses of radiation but some patients find it claustrophobic. MRI can't be used in patients with metallic foreign bodies such as cardiac pacemakers because of the effect of the magnetic field. MRI is useful in detecting various brain and spinal cord pathology. Magnetic resonance angiography (MRA) and magnetic resonance venogram (MRV) are also widely used to demonstrate abnormalities in intracranial blood vessels.

➤ Angiography: is still considered the 'gold standard' for imaging the intracranial blood vessels. However, it is mainly used as a treatment tool, for example in coiling aneurysms.

➤ Single-photon emission computerised tomography (SPECT) and positron emission tomography (PET) are of limited use in routine clinical practice.

NEUROPHYSIOLOGY

➤ Electroencephalogram (EEG): *see* p. 67.
➤ Nerve conduction study (NCS): by electrical stimulation of different peripheral nerves, it is possible to measure both sensory and motor function of these nerves. They are usually used in the assessment of peripheral neuropathy to differentiate between axonal and demyelinating neuropathy and to diagnose nerve entrapment.
➤ Electromyography (EMG): a fine needle inserted directly into a muscle to look for spontaneous activity and motor unit potential. EMG can be helpful in:
  ➣ assessment of peripheral neuropathy to differentiate between axonal and demyelinating neuropathy
  ➣ assessment of neuromuscular disorders such as myasthenia gravis (MG)
  ➣ demonstrating fibrillation potentials, for example in motor neurone disease (MND).

LUMBAR PUNCTURE AND CEREBROSPINAL FLUID

➤ Lumbar puncture (LP) is one of the most commonly used investigations in neurology. It is usually indicated in acute conditions such as acute headache or patients with a possible diagnosis of meningitis or encephalitis. It is also used in investigating patients with possible multiple sclerosis (MS) or any other inflammatory CNS disease.
➤ LP is contraindicated in patients with symptoms or signs attributable to raised intracranial pressure as this could lead to tentorial herniation and coning (*see* Chapter 16, p. 51).
➤ Routinely the cerebrospinal fluid (CSF) is analysed for protein, cells and glucose. Spectrophotometry looking for blood

breakdown products is indicated in suspected subarachnoid haemorrhage. Checking for oligoclonal bands is used to help to diagnose MS.

➤ The most common complication of LP is 'post-LP headache', which results from a reduction in intracranial pressure. The headache is worse on sitting or standing and usually resolves spontaneously within 7–10 days.

PART II

Neurological signs

CHAPTER 13

Cranial nerve disorders

OLFACTORY (1ST) NERVE
➤ Rarely examined in neurological practice. Anosmia (loss of sense of smell) is usually due to nasal problems. Head trauma is another cause.

OPTIC (2ND) NERVE
➤ The optic nerve disorders could be divided as following:
  ➢ pupil abnormalities
  ➢ visual field defects
  ➢ optic disc disorders.

Pupil abnormalities
➤ The optic nerve carries the afferent limb of the pupillary light reflex.
➤ Relative afferent pupillary defect (RAPD) is tested by the swinging light test (swing the light from one pupil to the other every second or two). Normal pupils constrict every time they are exposed to light. In afferent pupillary defect (APD) the pupil dilates instead when exposed to light. RAPD indicates optic nerve disease – usually optic neuritis in patients with MS.
➤ Horner's syndrome is another pupil abnormality that is encountered in clinical practice. However, Horner's syndrome

is *not* due to an optic nerve lesion but to a lesion in the sympathetic pathway. Clinically the patient presents with unilateral incomplete ptosis with no evidence of abnormal eye movement. Pupil is small and reacts to light and accommodation. Other features include enophthalmos (eye appears sunken) and lack of sweating of the face on the side of the lesion. The lesion in Horner's syndrome could occur at several sites: the hypothalamus, medulla, cervical cord or sympathetic chain. Causes of Horner's syndrome are:
- idiopathic
- Pancoast's syndrome as a result of apical lung malignancy
- trauma or surgery such as thyroid surgery
- thoracic outlet syndrome
- painful Horner's syndrome could be associated with migraine and carotid artery dissection
- other causes include syringomyelia, nasopharyngeal cancer and lateral medullary syndrome.
➤ Other pupillary defects *not* related to optic nerves (the site of pathology is not known) are:
- Argyll Robertson pupil is a rare classical neurological sign. It is a small irregular pupil reacting to accommodation but not to light, due to syphilis or diabetes.
- Adie's pupil is a unilateral dilated pupil not reacting to light (or sluggish reaction) in young or middle-aged women. Holmes–Adie syndrome is a combination of Adie's pupil and reduced or absent tendon reflexes.

Visual field defects
➤ The visual pathway includes the following:
- retina and optic nerve
- optic chiasm
- optic tract reaching lateral geniculate body
- optic radiation through parietal and temporal lobes
- visual cortex in the occipital lobe.
➤ Bitemporal hemianopia: visual field assessment showing evidence of impairment of both temporal fields as a result

of a lesion in the optic chiasma. Pituitary tumours are the main cause of optic chiasma lesions. Other causes include craniopharyngioma, meningioma and a large internal carotid artery aneurysm.

➤ Homonymous hemianopia: visual field assessment shows evidence of impairment of the temporal field on one side and the nasal field on the other side as a result of an optic tract lesion (behind the optic chiasma). The visual field defect in this case is on the contralateral side of the lesion (e.g. a lesion in the *right* posterior optic tract causes *left* homonymous hemianopia). Causes of optic tract lesions include cerebrovascular disease, such as occipital infarction, or haemorrhage. Other causes include tumours. The visual loss could be only in the quadrant of the visual field if the lesion is in the temporal lobe (superior quadrantanopia) or parietal lobe (inferior quadrantanopia).

Optic disc swelling (papilloedema)

➤ Papilloedema is an optic disc swelling due to raised intracranial pressure; therefore, optic disc swelling is a more correct term.

➤ Papilloedema causes absent venous pulsation and blurring of optic disc margin with or without haemorrhages or exudates.

➤ Causes of papilloedema include:
  ➤ Increased intracranial pressure that could be due to brain tumours, cerebrovenous sinus thrombosis (CVST) or cerebral abscess.
  ➤ If the patient is a young, obese woman then the likely diagnosis is idiopathic (benign) intracranial hypertension.
  ➤ Other rare causes include malignant hypertension and cavernous sinus thrombosis.

➤ Optic neuritis (papillitis) is another cause of optic disc swelling and is defined as acute inflammation of the optic nerve. MS is a common cause of optic neuritis. Retrobulbar optic neuritis causes inflammation of the optic disc with acute visual loss and a normal-looking optic disc.

➤ Optic neuritis causes visual loss, central scotoma, retro-orbital pain and a relative afferent pupillary defect. Papilloedema causes peripheral visual field constriction (visual acuity is usually normal until a very late stage). Patients may report headache and pupils are normal.

Optic atrophy
➤ The optic disc is pale with sharp margins.
➤ Causes of optic atrophy include:
  ➢ MS in young patients
  ➢ ischaemic optic neuropathy in older patients
  ➢ other causes include optic nerve compression, Leber's hereditary optic neuropathy, toxins (tobacco and methyl alcohol) and nutritional deficiencies (vitamins B_1 and B_{12}).
➤ Secondary optic atrophy is due to long-standing papilloedema. The discs appear pale with ill-defined disc margins.

OCULOMOTOR (3RD) NERVE
➤ The 3rd nerve nucleus is located in the midbrain. The nerve runs parallel to posterior communicating arteries and then passes through the cavernous sinus and enters the orbit through the superior orbital fissure.
➤ The oculomotor nerve supplies all muscles of the eye (medial rectus, superior rectus, inferior rectus and inferior oblique) except the lateral rectus (6th nerve) and superior oblique (4th nerve). It also supplies the levator palpebrae muscle and carries the parasympathetic fibres to the pupil (efferent limb of the pupillary light reflex).
➤ Patients usually present with partial or complete ptosis with eye deviation laterally (down and out) and impaired response to light and accommodation with or without pupillary dilatation.
➤ Causes of 3rd nerve palsy include:
  ➢ Ischaemic (microvascular) – usually painless with pupillary sparing in patients with diabetes and/or hypertension. Spontaneous recovery within 3–4 months is the usual outcome.
  ➢ Surgical causes – posterior communicating artery aneurysm (painful) or brainstem tumour.

➢ MS and migraine rarely cause isolated 3rd nerve palsy.

➢ A lesion in the superior orbital fissure or cavernous sinus such as metastasis, sphenoid wing meningioma, nasopharyngeal carcinoma, carotid siphon aneurysm or cavernous sinus thrombosis.

➢ Basal meningeal lesion as a result of infection (tuberculosis or fungal), carcinomatous, neurosarcoid or direct spread from nasopharyngeal tumour.

➢ Tentorial herniation and coning (*see* Chapter 16, p. 51).

TROCHLEAR (4TH) NERVE

➤ Isolated 4th nerve palsy is very rare in clinical practice and is usually due to head trauma. Other causes include ischaemia (microvascular) in patients with diabetes and/or hypertension.

➤ The 4th nerve supplies the superior oblique, which suppresses the adducted eye.

➤ Patients with 4th nerve palsy present with vertical diplopia, which is corrected by tilting the head.

➤ It can be tricky to see 4th nerve palsy in patients with 3rd nerve palsy. With 3rd nerve palsy the patient would not be able to adduct the affected eye; therefore, when asked to move the eye downwards the eye will rotate inwards if the 4th nerve is intact.

TRIGEMINAL (5TH) NERVE

➤ The 5th nerve nucleus is located in the pons. The nerve provides sensory supply to the face:

➢ ophthalmic (V1) – supplies the forehead to the vertex and the cornea

➢ maxillary (V2) – supplies the cheek

➢ mandibular (V3) – supplies the lower jaw but *not* the angle of the jaw.

➤ The motor component of the 5th nerve supplies the masseter and temporalis muscles. V1 and V2 pass through the cavernous sinus.

➤ Any pathology affecting the brainstem, cerebellopontine angle or cavernous sinus could lead to sensory abnormalities on the face with absent corneal reflexes. Trigeminal motor function is very rarely affected.

ABDUCENT (6TH) NERVE

➤ The 6th nerve nucleus is located in the pons. The nerve passes through the cavernous sinus and enters the orbit through the superior orbital fissure to supply the lateral rectus muscle.
➤ Patients usually present with horizontally separated double vision on looking to the side (right or left), with limitation of abduction of the eye.
➤ Causes of 6th nerve palsy include:
➢ Ischaemic (microvascular) – usually in patients with diabetes and/or hypertension. Spontaneous recovery within 3–4 months is the usual outcome.
➢ The 6th nerve is vulnerable to an increase in intracranial pressure due to the long peripheral course of the nerve. This leads to a false localising sign (*see* list of papilloedema causes, p. 35).
➢ Brainstem lesions such as a tumour or demyelination (MS).
➢ If there is involvement of other cranial nerves such as 3rd and 5th, consider superior orbital fissure, cavernous sinus or basal meningeal lesion (*see* list of 3rd nerve palsy causes, p. 36).

FACIAL (7TH) NERVE

➤ The facial nerve is primarily motor and its nucleus is located in the pons. The nerve leaves the pons at the cerebellopontine angle to enter the internal auditory meatus and the facial canal. It supplies to the stapedius muscle before emerging from the skull through the stylomastoid foramen to supply the facial muscles. The facial nerve also supplies the lacrimal and parotid glands and the taste to the anterior two-thirds of the tongue.
➤ Due to the bilateral cortical innervation of the facial nerve nucleus there are two types of 7th nerve palsy: UMN type (contralateral weakness of the lower part of the face with forehead and eye closure relatively spared) and LMN type (ipsilateral weakness of the whole side of the face).

➤ The most common cause of UMN 7th nerve palsy is a hemisphere stroke.

➤ Bell's palsy is a common cause of LMN 7th nerve palsy. Patients usually present with facial weakness involving the whole side of the face. Examination shows difficulty raising the eyebrow and inability to shut the eye fully, Bell's phenomenon (turning of the eye upwards when the patient is asked to shut the eyes), difficulty with cheek blowing, obliteration of the nasolabial fold and droopy mouth. No investigation is required in Bell's palsy. There is spontaneous full recovery in more than 80% of patients. The role of steroids and acyclovir is still controversial. However, they are commonly used, especially if the patient is seen within 72 hours from the onset of the palsy. Protection of the cornea by using artificial tears is essential.

➤ Other causes of LMN 7th nerve palsy include cerebellopontine angle lesions such as acoustic neuroma, middle ear infection, parotid tumour, parotid gland or ear surgery, pontine lesions such as a tumour, and Ramsay Hunt syndrome (herpes zoster infection affecting the geniculate (facial) ganglion).

➤ Hyperacusis (sound heard abnormally loudly) could be a feature of 7th nerve palsy.

➤ Bilateral LMN lesion of the 7th nerve can be tricky to detect due to absence of asymmetry. Causes of bilateral LMN 7th nerve include Guillain–Barré syndrome (GBS), neurosarcoid and Lyme disease.

VESTIBULOCOCHLEAR (8TH) NERVE

➤ The 8th nerve nucleus is located in the pons. The nerve exits at the cerebellopontine angle and enters the internal auditory meatus. It connects the cochlea (cochlear nerve) and labyrinth, also known as vestibular body (vestibular nerve), with the CNS. The function of the nerve is to maintain balance and equilibrium (vestibular nerve) and hearing (cochlear nerve).

➤ Lesions in the cerebellopontine angle such as acoustic neuroma could present with deafness and loss of balance.

➤ Patients with hearing loss usually present to ear, nose and throat

(ENT) clinics. Patients with Ménière's disease usually present with deafness, tinnitus and episodic vertigo and vomiting.

➤ Other relatively common problems that could present to either neurology or ENT clinics are acute labyrinthitis (vestibular neuronitis) and benign paroxysmal positional vertigo:

➢ *Acute labyrinthitis (vestibular neuronitis)* – a sudden onset of rotatory vertigo, vomiting and loss of balance to the extent that patient may not able to walk. The severe symptoms usually resolve within days but full recovery could take several weeks.

➢ *Benign paroxysmal positional vertigo* – episodes of short-lived vertigo, usually for only a matter of seconds, in certain positions such as turning in bed. Spontaneous resolution of the symptoms is expected.

➤ Any brainstem pathology such as vascular or demyelination could impair the function of the 8th nerve.

GLOSSOPHARYNGEAL (9TH), VAGUS (10TH) AND HYPOGLOSSAL (12TH) NERVES

➤ The 9th nerve supplies the palate and the pharynx, the 10th nerve supplies the pharynx and larynx, and the 12th nerve supplies the tongue muscles.

➤ Bulbar palsy (a bilateral LMN lesion of the lower cranial nerves): wasted and atrophic tongue with fasciculation. Causes of bulbar palsy include:

➢ MND

➢ syringobulbia

➢ skull base lesion that is usually due to cancer

➢ brainstem tumour.

➤ Pseudobulbar palsy (bilateral UMN of the lower cranial nerves): small, slow-moving spastic tongue. Causes of pseudobulbar palsy include:

➢ extensive cerebrovascular disease causing bilateral ischaemia

➢ MND.

➤ A mixture of both bulbar and pseudobulbar palsy is usually caused by MND and leads to slow-moving, wasted and atrophic tongue with fasciculation.

➤ A brisk jaw reflex, spastic slurring, dysarthria and emotional lability are features of pseudobulbar palsy.

➤ A depressed jaw reflex and nasal speech are features of bulbar palsy.

➤ Swallowing is usually impaired in both bulbar and pseudobulbar palsies.

➤ A unilateral LMN lesion of the 12th nerve usually presents with unilateral wasting and fasciculation of the tongue and deviation of the tongue to one side. The tongue deviates towards the side the lesion. Causes of unilateral LMN lesion 12th nerve palsy include:

  ➢ basal meningitis due to cancer, lymphoma, tuberculosis or sarcoidosis

  ➢ syringobulbia

  ➢ foramen magnum tumour

  ➢ nasopharyngeal tumour.

ACCESSORY (11TH) NERVE

➤ The 11th nerve supplies the sternomastoid. The sternomastoid muscle turns the head in the *opposite* direction (e.g. weakness of twisting head to the *right* is due to weakness of the *left* sternomastid).

➤ Jugular foramen syndrome is a classic neurological syndrome of unilateral 10th and 11th nerve palsy causing poor movement of the soft palate with deviation of the uvula and weakness in twisting the head and shrugging of the shoulders. Causes of jugular foramen syndrome include:

  ➢ tumours such as neurofibroma, meningioma and glomus jugulare tumour

  ➢ carcinomatous infiltration

  ➢ neurosarcoid

  ➢ infection spreading from middle ear disease.

➤ The uvula deviates *away* from the side of the lesion. However, the deviation of the midline soft palate could be a better indicator than the uvula.

CHAPTER 14

Common neurological patterns

MONOPLEGIA AND/OR HEMIPLEGIA

➤ There is unilateral arm and/or leg weakness with increased tone and brisk reflexes. There is possible impairment of pinprick sensation over affected side and facial weakness (ipsilateral UMN lesion of 7th nerve).

➤ The causes of monoplegia/hemiplegia are:
  ➢ cerebrovascular disease (sudden onset)
  ➢ brain tumour (gradual onset)
  ➢ spinal cord lesion (gradual onset).

➤ The investigation of monoplegia and/or hemiplegia could include the following:
  ➢ brain CT and/or MRI
  ➢ spinal MRI
  ➢ assessment of vascular risk factors such as blood sugar and cholesterol.

➤ If there is loss of joint position and vibration sense on the monoparetic side and loss of pain and temperature on the opposite side to a certain sensory level (e.g. T10) then the diagnosis is Brown-Séquard syndrome. This is usually caused by spinal cord tumour or MS.

SPASTIC PARAPARESIS AND/OR QUADRIPARESIS

➤ Bilateral increased (spastic) tone with brisk reflexes, and upgoing plantars in the lower limbs. There is (possible) weakness, ankle clonus and sensory level. The upper limbs may show signs of an UMN lesion.
➤ Common causes:
  ➢ MS in young patients
  ➢ cervical spondylotic myelopathy in middle-aged and older patients
  ➢ spinal trauma
  ➢ spinal tumours (primary or metastatic)
  ➢ vascular causes such as spinal arteriovenous malformation and spinal ischaemia (anterior spinal artery syndrome).
➤ Rare causes:
  ➢ B_{12} deficiency
  ➢ thoracic cord meningioma in middle-aged women
  ➢ MND
  ➢ hereditary spastic paraplegia
  ➢ tropical spastic paraplegia
  ➢ parasagittal meningioma
  ➢ syringomyelia.
➤ The investigation of spastic paraparesis and/or quadriparesis could include the following:
  ➢ brain MRI
  ➢ spine MRI
  ➢ CSF analysis – looking particularly for oligoclonal bands.
  ➢ other specific investigations if there is clear indication to the cause (e.g. NCS and/or EMG in MND, checking vitamin B_{12}).

PERIPHERAL NEUROPATHY

➤ Predominantly sensory peripheral neuropathy – there is reduction in pinprick sensation in the glove and stocking distribution. Also there is impairment in vibration and joint position sense. Ankle jerks may be absent.
➤ The causes of predominantly sensory peripheral neuropathy are:
  ➢ diabetes

- vitamin B deficiency (thiamine and B_{12}), especially in alcoholics
- paraneoplastic neuropathy
- drugs such as antituberculosis drugs (isoniazid and ethambutol) and chemotherapeutic agents (cisplantinum and vincristine)
- amyloidosis and chronic renal failure
- idiopathic especially in older patients
- paraproteinaemic neuropathy (mixed sensory and motor neuropathy).

➤ Predominantly motor peripheral neuropathy – bilateral generalised weakness that is more marked distally with absent jerks and mild impairment of pinprick, joint position and vibration sense.

➤ The causes of predominantly motor peripheral neuropathy are:
  - GBS
  - chronic inflammatory demyelinating polyradiculoneuropathy (CIDP)
  - Charcot–Marie–Tooth disease (CMT)
  - porphyria
  - lead poisoning.

➤ The investigations could include:
  - NCS and/or EMG – important to confirm the diagnosis and to determine whether there is axonal neuropathy or demyelinating neuropathy
  - CSF analysis – looking particularly for high protein (demyelinating neuropathy)
  - blood sugar
  - full blood count and erythrocyte sedimentation rate (ESR)
  - liver function test
  - vitamin B_{12}
  - vasculitic screen
  - paraprotein screen
  - special investigations such as paraneoplastic antibodies and sural nerve biopsy may be needed in some patients.

ATAXIA

➤ Patients usually present with loss of balance. Examination may show ataxic gait (wide-based gait), difficulty performing the heel-to-toe walking (drunken gait), nystagmus, dysarthria, abnormal finger-to-nose test, abnormal heel-to-shin test, intention tremor (worse on approaching the target), and dysdiadochokinesia (breakdown of rhythmic, rapid alternating movements such as rapid pronation and supination movements of one hand on the other one).

➤ The causes of ataxic syndrome are:
  ➤ MS
  ➤ alcoholic cerebellar degeneration (usually gait ataxia)
  ➤ drugs such as anticonvulsants (phenytoin and carbamazepine) and lithium
  ➤ stroke – either ischaemic or haemorrhagic
  ➤ paraneoplastic syndrome (usually with lung or breast cancer)
  ➤ spinocerebellar ataxia (genetic ataxia)
  ➤ idiopathic cerebellar ataxia
  ➤ Friedreich's ataxia (pes cavus, absent ankle jerks, upgoing planters and scoliosis)
  ➤ posterior fossa tumours
  ➤ hypothyroidism.

➤ The speed of the onset of ataxia, the age of onset and family history can give clues as to the cause of the ataxia.

➤ The investigation of ataxic syndrome should be tailored to the possible cause but could include:
  ➤ brain MRI
  ➤ CSF analysis – looking particularly for oligoclonal bands
  ➤ anticonvulsant blood level
  ➤ paraneoplastic antibodies
  ➤ genetic testing for spinocerebellar ataxia or Friedreich's ataxia
  ➤ NCS and/or EMG.

CHAPTER 15

Peripheral nerve lesions

MEDIAN NERVE PALSY

➤ Median nerve palsy is commonly due to entrapment of the nerve at the wrist (carpal tunnel syndrome).

➤ Clinically patients usually present with sensory symptoms such as paraesthesia affecting the hand and possibly radiating up to the elbow. The symptoms are worse at night and relieved by shaking the hands.

➤ On examination there is sensory loss over the palmar aspects of the thumb, index and middle fingers and the lateral half of the ring finger. Less commonly the patient could have wasting of the thenar eminence and weakness of abductor pollicis brevis of the hand leading to weakness of flexion and opposition of the thumb. Tinel's test (percussion over the palmar side of the wrist to produce paraesthesia over the median nerve distribution) and Phalen's test (dorsiflexing the wrist for a minute to produce paraesthesia over the median nerve distribution) may be positive.

➤ Carpal tunnel syndrome is more common in females as women have a narrower cross-sectional area in the carpal tunnel.

➤ The causes of carpal tunnel syndrome are:
  ➤ idiopathic (common in neurology clinics!)

- ➤ endocrine disorders such as hypothyroidism, diabetes and acromegaly
- ➤ rheumatological diseases such as rheumatoid arthritis and osteoarthritis
- ➤ others (pregnancy, oral contraceptive pills and amyloidosis).
- ➤ Upper limb NCS helps in confirming the diagnosis.
- ➤ Diuretics, wrist splints and local steroid injection could help in relieving the symptoms but surgical decompression may be needed.

ULNAR NERVE PALSY

- ➤ Ulnar nerve palsy is commonly due to entrapment of the nerve at the elbow.
- ➤ Clinically, patients usually present with sensory symptoms affecting the little finger, the medial half of the ring finger and the medial side of the hand (to the level of the wrist) and weakness in the handgrip. Examination shows impairment of pinprick sensation over the little finger, the medial half of the ring finger and the medial side of the hand. There could be generalised wasting and weakness of the small muscles of the hand, which is more prominent in the first dorsal interosseous muscle with sparing of the thenar eminence. There may also be a claw hand (hyperextension at the metacarpophalangeal joints and flexion at the interphalangeal joints of the little and ring fingers).
- ➤ If the sensory signs extend to the elbow then the lesion is at C8/ T1 level.
- ➤ The causes of ulnar nerve entrapment at the elbow are:
  - ➤ chronic compression due to old fracture, or dislocation at the elbow or osteoarthritic change
  - ➤ acute compression due to fracture or after general anaesthesia
  - ➤ occupational (e.g. painters, bricklayers and secretaries)
  - ➤ part of mononeuritis multiplex.
- ➤ NCS is important to confirm the diagnosis and determine the level of the lesion.

➤ The treatment is usually conservative by avoidance, if possible, of further compression. Ulnar nerve decompression or transposition could be considered in severe cases.

RADIAL NERVE PALSY

➤ There is weakness in dorsiflexion of the wrist (wrist drop) and the patient is unable to straighten the fingers due to weakness of the finger extensors at the metacarpophalangeal joints.

➤ If the patient's wrist is passively extended the patient will be able to straighten the fingers at the interphalangeal joints but not at the metacarpophalangeal joints as the interossei and lumbricals are functioning normally.

➤ The extensor digitorum, extensor indicis and extensor carpi ulnaris are the main wrist extensors and are all supplied by the radial nerve.

➤ Abduction and adduction of the fingers may appear weak unless they are tested when the wrist is rested flat.

➤ Due to overlap in the sensory supply by the median, ulnar and radial nerves, only a small area of impaired sensation in the skin over the first dorsal interosseous muscle is affected in radial nerve palsy.

➤ The triceps and brachioradialis may be affected if the lesion of the radial nerve is high (above middle third of the humerus).

➤ The causes of radial nerve palsy are:
  ➤ Acute compression at the 'spiral groove' after a general anaesthetic or being unconscious (Saturday night palsy – this tends to occur in people who are drunk as they go to sleep with the arm hanging over the side of an armchair. The tricep is spared).
  ➤ Fractured shaft of the humerus.
  ➤ Crutch trauma at the level of the axilla (rare).

➤ NCS is important to confirm the diagnosis and determine the level of the lesion.

➤ The treatment is usually conservative with a wrist splint and physiotherapy. Full recovery is usual in the case of acute compression. The outcome is variable after a humerus fracture.

COMMON PERONEAL NERVE PALSY

➤ There is weakness in dorsiflexion of the ankle and eversion of foot (foot drop). There is possible reduction in pinprick sensation over the lateral aspect of the calf and the dorsum of the foot. Ankle jerk is preserved. The dorsiflexion (extensor hallucis longus of the big toe) can be weak; this can be tested by asking the patient to move the toe against resistance.

➤ The common peroneal nerve has two branches, the superficial and the deep branch. If the lesion is below the origin of the superficial branch the sensory changes will be confined to a small area of the dorsum area between the big and the second toes.

➤ Patient could have a steppage gait as seen by lifting the foot high during walking to avoid scraping the toes and foot slapping.

➤ Injury to the common peroneal nerve usually occurs at the level of the fibula as a result of trauma or compression.

➤ Other causes of foot drop are:
  ➤ L5 root lesion if the inversion of the ankle is also weak. This is usually painful.
  ➤ Sciatic nerve lesion if there is weakness of toe plantar flexion and loss of ankle jerk (tibial nerve involvement).
  ➤ Could be part of a generalised neurological problem such as peripheral neuropathy, MND (ankle reflexes will be brisk with no sensory signs) or cauda equina lesion.

➤ NCS is important to confirm the diagnosis.

➤ Treatment is usually conservative with an ankle splint.

CHAPTER 16

Coma (unconsciousness)

- Consciousness depends on the reticular activating system in the brainstem being intact.
- Consciousness includes both arousal and awareness.
- Avoid using terms such as 'stuporose' or 'obtunded'.
- The causes of coma include the following:
  - CNS infection (meningitis and encephalitis).
  - Electrolyte abnormalities.
  - Metabolic causes such as hypoglycaemia, diabetic ketoacidosis, hypoxia, liver and renal failure.
  - Seizures.
  - Cerebral haemorrhage (intracerebral and subarachnoid haemorrhage).
  - Poisons and drug overdose such as alcohol and opiate toxicity.
  - Tentorial herniation and coning – a mass lesion in the brain pushes the cerebral hemisphere through the tentorial hiatus (tentorial herniation), causing the brainstem and cerebellum to be pushed downwards and become impacted in the foramen magnum (coning).
  - Head injury.
- The Glasgow Coma Scale (GCS) is vital in assessing and reporting a patient's level of consciousness. The GCS has the

following components – the patient's score should be recorded, for example, as 9 (E3M4V2):

➢ *Eye opening (E)*
  • Spontaneous = 4
  • To speech = 3
  • To pain = 2
  • None = 1

➢ *Motor response (M)*
  • Obeys commands = 6
  • Localises to pain = 5
  • Flexion withdrawal to pain = 4
  • Abnormal flexion of upper limbs = 3
  • Abnormal extension = 2
  • None = 1

➢ *Best verbal response (V)*
  • Oriented = 5
  • Disoriented = 4
  • Inappropriate word = 3
  • Incomprehensible = 2
  • None = 1

➤ Management includes:
  ➢ ABC – maintain clear airway, assess breathing and support the circulation by monitoring the blood pressure, pulse and establishing an IV line.
  ➢ Blood tests – full blood count, urea and electrolytes and blood glucose. Also drug screening (e.g. paracetamol level) and arterial blood gas if clinically indicated.
  ➢ Look for signs of trauma and meningism.
  ➢ Check the size of the pupils (small pupils could be due to opiate overdose).
  ➢ History from family or any eyewitness. If possible, contact the general practitioner.
  ➢ Brain CT, EEG and LP if clinically indicated.
  ➢ Treat the underlying cause – for example, give IV glucose in hypoglycaemia or anticonvulsants in seizures.

PART III

Neurological problems and diseases – the big five

CHAPTER 17

Headache

- ➤ Headache is the most common neurological problem that neurologists deal with in outpatient clinics.
- ➤ You could think of causes of headache in the following way:
  - ➤ Benign (green light!) – most causes of headache are benign (tension headache, migraine, overused medication headache, cluster headache, trigeminal neuralgia and post-traumatic headache).
  - ➤ Serious (amber light!) – headache could be the main symptom of some serious diseases. Missing or delaying the diagnosis could lead to permanent loss of vision (giant cell arteritis and idiopathic intracranial hypertension).
  - ➤ Dangerous (red light!) – headache could be a symptom of dangerous diseases such as subarachnoid haemorrhage (*see* Chapter 19, p. 78) or meningitis (*see* Chapter 22, p. 102). However, contrary to general belief, brain tumours rarely present with headache only.
- ➤ The classic teaching indicates that morning headaches which increase with coughing and are associated with vomiting are due to raised intracranial pressure. However, in clinical practice migraine tends to be more associated with such symptoms while patients with raised intracranial pressure usually have new onset,

mild and short-lived featureless headaches. Focal symptoms and signs may or may not present.

➤ Patients can have more than one type of benign headache – for example, tension *and* migraine headache.

➤ The diagnosis of benign headaches is based on good history taking. Examination and scans rarely help apart from reassuring the patient and the doctor!

TENSION HEADACHE

➤ Tension headache is the most common type of headache.

➤ The headache is usually generalised and daily. Patients may describe it as a tight band around the head or as the head being in a vice. There are no gastrointestinal or visual symptoms associated with the headache.

➤ Headache does not interfere with sleep.

➤ Patients may have underlying anxiety or depression.

➤ Patients need reassurance that nothing sinister is causing the headache. Amitriptyline is widely used. Although a brain scan is not indicated it is increasingly being used for reassurance.

MIGRAINE HEADACHE

➤ Migraine headache is more common in women and young people.

➤ The headache is episodic and usually lasts from several hours to 3 days.

➤ The unilateral throbbing headache could be preceded by aura that can last for 20–30 minutes. Pain behind the eye is common. Headache is made worse with movement.

➤ The most common type of aura is visual where patients experience flashing lights or zigzag lines. Other types of aura – such as paraesthesia in the hand spreading upwards to involve the lips and the tongue, unilateral weakness or speech difficulties – are less common.

➤ Nausea, vomiting, photophobia (dislike of light) and phonophobia (dislike of sound) are associated with migraine. Sleep helps in relieving the headache.

➤ Contrary to public belief, finding a specific trigger factor for migraine, such as eating cheese, is not common in clinical practice. However, menstruation is commonly reported as a trigger factor.

➤ Patients need a full explanation of the diagnosis and different treatment strategies. Reassurance that nothing sinister is causing the headache is important. Again, brain scan is not indicated in the majority of cases but it is increasingly being used for reassurance.

➤ The treatment of migraine includes the following:
  ➤ Avoiding trigger factors (if you find one!).
  ➤ Treating the acute attacks with simple analgesia such as paracetamol or aspirin. Or simple analgesia combined with antiemetics, such as Migraleve. If these fail, triptans ($5HT_1$ agonists) are commonly used and are available as tablets, nasal spray and subcutaneous injections.
  ➤ Preventive treatment should be considered if patients experience frequent attacks (more than two per month). Propranolol, amitriptyline, pizotifen and topiramate are commonly used.

MEDICATION OVERUSE HEADACHE

➤ Medication overuse headache is a chronic daily headache (dull or throbbing pain) resulting from taking analgesia (especially those containing codeine) almost on a daily basis to treat tension or migraine headache. The headache is transiently relieved by analgesia.

➤ It is important to explain to patients the harmful effects of overusing analgesia. Preventative treatment for headache such as amitriptyline should be introduced and the analgesia should be stopped gradually or abruptly (although this is easier said than done!).

CLUSTER HEADACHE

➤ Cluster headache is uncommon. It predominantly affects men and occurs in clusters (once or twice daily, for 4–8 weeks, once every year or two).

➤ The headache usually lasts from half an hour to 2 hours, mainly at night. It tends to occur at the same time each day – for example, at 1 a.m. each day for the whole length of the cluster.

➤ It is a unilateral excruciating pain around the eye associated with watering and redness of the eye, nasal blockage and, occasionally, Horner's syndrome.

➤ The treatment of cluster headaches includes the following:
  ➤ Treating the acute attacks with sumatriptan subcutaneous injection ($5HT_1$ agonist) or by high-flow oxygen.
  ➤ Preventative treatment should be given until the cluster is over. Pizotifen, verapamil, topiramate and steroids are used.

TRIGEMINAL NEURALGIA

➤ Trigeminal neuralgia usually affects people above the age of 40 years. It is believed that trigeminal neuralgia is caused by irritation of the 5th nerve by an ectatic blood vessel. However, in younger patients it may be associated with MS.

➤ Patient presents with severe unilateral pain lasting for seconds (like electric shock or needle stabs) over the area supplied by one of the branches of the 5th nerve, usually the maxillary or mandibular.

➤ Patient usually experiences several attacks a day and may complain of dull aching pains between the episodes.

➤ Talking, eating, drinking, shaving and washing the face may trigger the attacks.

➤ The treatment of trigeminal neuralgia includes the following:
  ➤ Anticonvulsants – carbamazepine is the usual first choice. Phenytoin, lamotrigine and gabapentin are also used.
  ➤ Surgical treatment includes glycerol injection of the 5th nerve and microvascular decompression.

POST-TRAUMATIC HEADACHE

➤ Following any type of head injury, including minor ones, patients may experience headaches for several weeks or months.
➤ The headache usually starts within 2 weeks of the injury.
➤ The headache could be part of post-traumatic (concussion) syndrome where patients can experience other symptoms such as lack of concentration, poor memory and dizziness.
➤ Patients may need reassurance with a brain scan.
➤ Amitriptyline is widely used as treatment.

GIANT CELL (TEMPORAL) ARTERITIS

➤ Giant cell arteritis is a disease that affects older people. Patients present with pain and tenderness at the temple. Patients find it difficult to brush their hair. Non-specific symptoms such as feeling generally unwell are common. Examination can show tenderness around the temple and the lack of pulsation of the temporal artery.
➤ ESR (usually > 60) and temporal artery biopsy are the investigations of choice.
➤ Patients should be treated immediately with oral steroid to avoid permanent loss of vision due to infarction of the optic nerve. Headache settling within a day from starting treatment is diagnostic. Patients will normally need a maintenance dose of steroid for some years.

IDIOPATHIC INTRACRANIAL HYPERTENSION

➤ The patient in this case is typically an obese young woman presenting with headache and blurred vision.
➤ Examination shows bilateral papilloedema.
➤ Brain scan is normal and CSF pressure is high but with normal constituents. CTV or MRV to exclude CVST is essential.
➤ Patients should be treated promptly to avoid permanent loss of vision due to infarction of the optic nerve.
➤ The management includes the following:
  ➤ full and regular visual assessment including visual fields
  ➤ weight loss

➤ diuretics such as acetazolamide
➤ if the vision deteriorates neurosurgical intervention is needed (lumboperitoneal shunting).

CHAPTER 18

Epilepsy

➤ Seizure is defined as an abnormal function of the brain as a result of abnormal paroxysmal neuronal discharge. Clinically, epilepsy is defined as a tendency to have recurrent seizures (more than one unprovoked seizure).

➤ Epilepsy is a common neurological disease with an overall annual incidence of 50–120 per 100 000 of the population and prevalence rate of 4–10 per 1000 of the population.

➤ Epilepsy has bimodal age of onset with higher incidence in children and older people.

➤ Male and female are similarly affected.

CAUSES

➤ Seizure is considered to be a symptom, not a disease. In 25% of epilepsy patients a specific cause will be identified. Brain tumour, cerebral infarction, cerebral haemorrhage, cerebral venous thrombosis and arteriovenous malformation could present with seizures. Head injury is an important cause of post-traumatic epilepsy. Seizures might be associated with other neurological diseases such as meningitis, encephalitis and neurodegenerative diseases. Alcohol, drugs, toxins, metabolic and biochemical disorders can all lead to seizures.

➤ Genetic factors also contribute to the aetiology of epilepsy. This could be as a single major locus or interaction of several loci with environmental factors.

SEIZURE TYPES

➤ Seizures are broadly classified as partial-onset or generalised. The seizure discharges originate from a localised part of the cerebral hemisphere in partial-onset seizures while in generalised seizures the discharges are simultaneous and involve both cerebral hemispheres. Partial-onset seizures may spread to involve the whole brain, leading to secondary generalisation.

Partial-onset seizures

➤ Partial-onset seizures may present with the following symptoms:
  ➤ Motor – rhythmic twitching or jerking of one part of the body opposite to the epileptic focus, such as fingers, toes or face, may spread to the rest of the body part (Jacksonian). Sustained tonic or dystonic movement of one limb and the head with eyes turning could be another feature. This can last for seconds or minutes.
  ➤ Sensory – tingling or numbness affecting one part of the body. Visual symptoms such as flashing lights may occur.
  ➤ High cortical function – dysphasic symptoms, disturbance of memory in a form of flashbacks, and déjà vu are well-recognised symptoms. Being in dreamy states, fear, anger, irritability, illusions of size, shape, weight, distance or sound may be features of a seizure. Visual, auditory, gustatory or olfactory symptoms can occur.
➤ Partial-onset seizures are called simple if consciousness is not impaired and complex if consciousness is impaired.
➤ Complex partial-onset seizures consist of three components:
  ➤ Aura – these are simple partial-onset seizures as described earlier (motor, sensory and high cortical function). They can be so short that patients would not be able to recall them.
  ➤ Automatism – a coordinated involuntary motor activity that occurred either during or after the seizure. This includes

fiddling movements with hands, lip smacking, chewing, emotional expression, humming, grunting and whistling.

➤ Impaired consciousness – can be in the form of an absence or motor arrest. The patient may appear vacant or glazed.

➤ The most common type of partial-onset seizures is temporal lobe epilepsy (60%), which usually presents with an epigastric sensation that rises up to the throat, high cortical function manifestations, auras, altered consciousness and automatism.

➤ Frontal lobe epilepsy represents 30% of partial-onset seizures and usually presents initially with deviation of the head and eyes to one side, and is associated with jerking of the arm on the same side. This may be followed by paralysis of the arm (Todd's paralysis). It can also cause complex or bizarre automatisms.

➤ Parietal lobe seizures can present with sensory symptoms, and occipital seizures may cause visual symptoms such as visual hallucinations with impairment in sensations of colours, shapes and patterns. Both parietal and occipital epilepsy are uncommon.

Generalised seizures

➤ Generalised seizures could be divided into three main types:

➤ *Tonic–clonic seizures* – patients may cry out then fall, becoming rigid with jaw clenching, breath holding and froth coming from the mouth (tonic phase). This is followed by the clonic phase: rhythmic clonic jerking of the limbs, neck and back followed by tongue biting and urinary incontinence. On coming round patients are usually confused, irritable, drowsy with headaches and muscle pain and tend to go to sleep in what is called the post-ictal stage. As a result of the seizures patients may sustain injuries. The tonic phase could last for seconds; the clonic phase for minutes; while the post-ictal stage could go on for hours. Sometimes there is no tonic phase (clonic seizures) or no clonic phase (tonic seizures). Also, patients may suddenly collapse as a result of losing muscle tone associated with loss of consciousness (atonic seizures).

➢ *Absence seizures* – usually occur in children and have two types, typical and atypical. In typical absences there is a sudden, momentary loss of contact with the surroundings, possibly with some minor jerking in the eyelids. These attacks may occur several times a day without the child's awareness and may present as learning difficulties. Atypical absences, which are more common, tend to occur in children with brain damage. They tend to be prolonged and are associated with dropping to the ground, leading to injuries.

➢ *Myoclonic seizures* – these are sudden, brief jerks that affect the upper limb and are with or without loss of consciousness. They may precede a generalised tonic–clonic seizure, often in the morning and occur in late childhood. This can form part of what is called juvenile myoclonic epilepsy.

EPILEPTIC SYNDROMES

➤ Patients who present with certain symptoms and signs could be classified as having epileptic syndrome. The classification of the syndromes is based on clinical history, EEG manifestations and aetiology.

➤ The epileptic syndromes are divided into idiopathic, when no cause is known, or symptomatic, when a cause is found. Cryptogenic epilepsies are defined as syndromes that are believed to be symptomatic but no aetiology has been identified.

DIFFERENTIAL DIAGNOSIS

Syncope

➤ Syncope is the most common cause of loss of consciousness.

➤ Syncope is a result of an abrupt and transient drop in blood pressure leading to a reduction in the brain's blood flow.

➤ A typical attack starts with the pre-syncopal phase when the patient feels nauseated, clammy and sweaty combined with blurring and loss of vision, dizziness, lightheadedness and tinnitus. The patient appears pale and sweaty, which is followed by loss of consciousness and falling to the floor. The patient usually looks floppy with eyes rolled up. When the patient regains consciousness they become flushed and may feel unwell, drowsy and slightly confused for a short time. Urinary incontinence is uncommon but could happen, especially if the bladder was full at the time. Tongue biting is rare. Syncopal attacks commonly occur in a standing position but can also occur in a sitting position. The patient may appear stiff and a few myoclonic jerks can lead to confusion with epileptic seizure.

➤ Vasovagal syncope and postural hypotension are common causes of syncope. Cardiac disorders such as arrhythmias or structural lesions can present with syncope. Cardiac syncope tends to occur in any position, particularly during exercise and emotional situations.

Non-epileptic attack disorder

➤ Non-epileptic attack disorder or psychogenic non-epileptic seizures (previously known as pseudoseizures) is commonly misdiagnosed as epilepsy. It is more common in women and usually starts in adolescence or early adulthood.

➤ A history of emotional trauma such as sexual abuse is common, as well as a history of abnormal illness behaviour such as recurrent unexplained abdominal pain.

➤ The attacks can be divided into two types: fall down, lie still unresponsive and convulsive; fall down with coarse alternating movement (usually) or thrashing (less common). Pelvic thrusting is characteristic but rather uncommon. Patients may resist any attempts to open their eyes during the attacks. Patients may recover rapidly from the attacks or recovery may take a prolonged period of time, and they may be very tearful.

Others

➤ Panic attacks, hyperventilation, transient ischaemic attacks (TIAs), hypoglycaemic episodes, migraine and movement disorders such as tics and chorea can all be misdiagnosed as epilepsy.

DIAGNOSIS

➤ The diagnosis of epilepsy is a *clinical* one and taking a proper history is crucial. Every effort must be made to get an eyewitness account of the seizure(s). Examination rarely helps but should be carried out to look for any abnormal neurological signs. Cardiological assessment and electrocardiogram (ECG) is essential, especially if syncope is suspected. Past medical history, family history of epilepsy and drug history are important.

➤ The following steps should be followed to get a proper history:

  ➤ *Events before the attack (from the patient)*
  - Number of attacks.
  - The duration of the attacks, the shortest and the longest attack.
  - The gap between the attacks (days, weeks or months).
  - The dates of the first and the last attack.
  - General health in the days before and on the day of the attack.
  - Precipitating factors such as changing position, stress and menstrual cycle.
  - Exact position just before the attack.
  - The time of the attack and whether it occurred during sleep.
  - Warning symptoms such as aura or palpitations.

  ➤ *Events during the attack (from the eyewitness)*
  - Change in colour.
  - Breathing pattern.
  - Abnormal movements.
  - Tone (rigid or floppy).
  - Duration of the attack.

  ➤ *Events after the attack (from the patient and the eyewitness)*
  - Tongue biting.
  - Incontinence.
  - Confusion.
  - Headache.
  - Muscle aches and pain.
  - Feeling sleepy and drowsy.
  - Any abnormal behaviour.

INVESTIGATION

➤ Patients may need an ECG or a full cardiological assessment if the history or examination is suggestive of a cardiac disorder.

EEG

➤ EEG is very commonly used (and abused) in clinical practice in patients with suspected epilepsy. The EEG should *only* be used to *support a clinical diagnosis* of epilepsy.

➤ A normal EEG does not exclude the diagnosis of epilepsy, as only 30%–40% of patients with epilepsy have epileptiform discharges on a routine (inter-ictal) EEG. An abnormal routine EEG is not in itself diagnostic of epilepsy, as up to 4% of subjects with abnormal EEGs do not have a history of epilepsy.

➤ EEG is usually a poor guide to seizure control or to the likelihood of seizure relapse.

➤ A routine EEG includes a period of activation by overbreathing for 3 minutes and photic stimulation. Sleep EEG could show epileptiform discharges in up to 70%–80% of patients with a clinical diagnosis of epilepsy and therefore it could be requested when a routine EEG is normal or borderline abnormal.

➤ The EEG may show focal or generalised spike or spike-and-wave activity, and therefore helps in localising an epileptogenic focus, which, in turn, leads to the classification of the epilepsy, such as three per second generalised spike-and-wave discharge in typical absence seizures. Also, specific EEG abnormalities are found in certain epilepsy syndromes.

➤ Continuous or intermittent EEG is needed in monitoring patients with status epilepticus, both as a diagnostic tool and to monitor the treatment, especially if general anaesthesia was required.

➤ Ambulatory EEG and video-EEG telemetry are useful in monitoring prolonged attacks ranging from 1 to 5 days, and are especially helpful in patients with frequent attacks and diagnostic difficulties (patients with non-epileptic attack disorders). Also, they are used to localise seizures prior to considering any surgical treatment.

Neuroimaging
➤ There have been great advances in neuroimaging over the last decade and this has helped to identify structural lesions causing seizures and epilepsy syndromes.
➤ MRI is the scan of choice and its superiority to CT is well established. However, CT of the brain can certainly help in identifying structural abnormalities such as tumours. MRI is needed in patients with partial-onset seizures and refractory epilepsy, and in patients in whom surgical treatment is under consideration, as it can highlight abnormalities such as hippocampal sclerosis.
➤ SPECT and PET are of limited use in routine clinical practice but can be used in specialised centres in pre-surgical workup and in research.

MANAGEMENT
➤ A diagnosis of epilepsy is a major event in patients' lives and can have a huge impact on their social life. Therefore, a full explanation of the diagnosis is essential. Patients should be given leaflets explaining the diagnosis and every effort should be taken to reassure the patients and encourage them to lead as normal a life as possible. However, general advice about driving, avoiding dangerous sports and not using dangerous and sharp tools should be discussed.

Anticonvulsants
➤ Anticonvulsants are the main treatment of epilepsy. Drug treatment is usually needed for at least 2–3 years and is sometimes lifelong. Therefore, patients should understand the nature of the treatment to increase their compliance. Most clinicians in the UK do not treat patients with a single seizure.
➤ There are general principles that need to be applied in using anticonvulsants. The aim of the treatment is freedom from seizures. The chosen drug should be introduced at a low dose and gradually increased to reach the standard dose. If seizures

are not controlled the dose should slowly be increased to the maximum tolerated, before changing to another drug. Patients should be treated with monotherapy if possible. However, combined therapy is needed in 10%–15% of patients with epilepsy.

➤ There are many anticonvulsants that can be used in clinical practice. The choice of medication usually depends on the type of epilepsy, although the majority of anticonvulsants can be used in both generalised and partial-onset seizures.

➤ *Carbamazepine* and *sodium valproate* are widely used in clinical practice as first-line treatments. Carbamazepine is indicated in patients with partial-onset seizures and should not be used in patients with absences and myoclonic seizures. It can cause skin rash in up to 10% of patients. Diplopia, headache, dizziness, nausea and vomiting are common side effects. Hyponatraemia is common but is usually of no clinical significance. *Oxcarbazepine*, which was introduced in the late 1990s, is an analogue of carbamazepine and has similar indications but fewer side effects. Sodium valproate is considered to be a broad-spectrum antiepileptic drug and particularly useful in idiopathic generalised epilepsies. However, it can cause tremor, weight gain, hair loss, amenorrhoea, polycystic ovarian syndrome and, rarely, hepatotoxicity, particularly in children. Thrombocytopenia and pancreatitis are rare side effects.

➤ *Lamotrigine* and *topiramate* are currently used as a first-line treatment for both partial-onset and generalised epilepsy. Skin rash is reported in 5% of patients taking lamotrigine. Headaches, drowsiness, ataxia, diplopia, insomnia, nausea and dizziness are also common side effects. Weight loss is common with topiramate and usually does not cause a problem to patients. The majority of the other side effects are related to the nervous system, such as dizziness, drowsiness, headaches, irritability, cognitive impairment and speech problems. Renal stones are a well-reported side effect.

➤ *Levetiracetam* was introduced in 2000 as an adjunctive therapy in adults with partial-onset seizures. It is now indicated as an adjunctive therapy in myoclonic seizures and as a monotherapy for partial-onset seizures. Somnolence, depression, dizziness and headache are the most common side effects. Psychosis is a well recognised but rare adverse event.

➤ *Gabapentin* and *vigabatrin* were used in the 1990s as an adjunctive treatment in patients with partial-onset epilepsy. However, gabapentin has been shown to be ineffective and is now commonly used for neuropathic pain, while vigabatrin has proven to cause visual field defects in up to 50% of patients and is rarely used.

➤ *Zonisamide, pregabalin* and *lacosamide* are the recent additions to the list of anticonvulsants and are indicated as an adjunctive therapy in partial-onset seizures. Dizziness, headache and drowsiness are common side effects. Zonisamide can cause somnolence, anorexia and weight loss while pregabalin can lead to weight gain.

➤ Other antiepileptic drugs (AEDs) such as *tiagabine, ethosuximide, piracetam* and *benzodiazepines* (*clobazam, clonazepam*) are occasionally used in clinical practice. Tiagabine is used as an adjunctive treatment in patients with partial-onset epilepsy not controlled with other anticonvulsants. The only use of ethosuximide is for children with absence seizures, while piracetam is used as an adjunctive treatment in adults with refractory myoclonus. Benzodiazepines can be used in treating patients with learning difficulties and refractory epilepsy.

➤ *Phenobarbitone* is one of the oldest anticonvulsants and is seldom used in developed countries due to its toxic side effects – mainly on cognition, mood and behaviour. *Primidone* is metabolised to phenobarbitone and has a similar toxic profile but no advantages over phenobarbitone.

➤ *Phenytoin* has been around since the 1930s. It is seldom used as a first-line treatment. Phenytoin requires monitoring of blood level and commonly causes acute and chronic toxic effects such as rash, hepatotoxicity, blood dyscrasias, drowsiness, tremor, ataxia, gum hyperplasia, acne, hirsutism, facial coarsening and cognitive difficulties.

➤ Drug interaction is an important issue to be considered in patients taking anticonvulsants and other drugs such as warfarin. Carbamazepine, oxcarbazepine, phenobarbitone, primidone, phenytoin and to some extent lamotrigine and topiramate are enzyme inducers, while sodium valproate is an enzyme inhibitor. Levetiracetam, gabapentin, vigabatrin, zonisamide, pregabalin, ethosuximide, piracetam and benzodiazepines have no significant drug interactions. Tiagabine's metabolism is faster in enzyme-induced patients.

➤ Measuring drug levels in the blood is of limited use – it is mainly used to check the patient's compliance or in case of carbamazepine or phenytoin toxicity.

➤ Stopping anticonvulsants can be discussed with the patient if they achieve seizure-freedom for at least 2 years. The risk of relapse is up to 40%. The decision to stop anticonvulsants is personal and the majority of the patients prefer to take the medication rather than risk losing their driving licence.

Surgical treatment

➤ Patients who are considered as being drug-resistant can be assessed for surgical treatment. This includes details of clinical history, brain MRI and sometimes SPECT or PET scans, neuropsychometry assessment and EEG including ambulatory or video telemetry if necessary.

➤ The type of surgical intervention depends on the type of epilepsy and the result of various pre-surgical investigations. Temporal lobe resection, extratemporal resection, hemispherectomy, corpus callosotomy and vagus nerve stimulation are all well-recognised surgical techniques, with temporal lobe resection being the most common operation.

➤ The results of surgical treatment are generally good in experienced centres, with 40%–87% of seizure-freedom.

➤ Surgical intervention could be part of early treatment in patients presenting with seizures and found to have a major structural abnormality such as a brain tumour or arteriovenous malformation.

MANAGEMENT OF TONIC–CLONIC STATUS EPILEPTICUS

➤ Tonic–clonic status epilepticus is a medical emergency and prompt treatment is required to prevent any long-term cerebral damage.

➤ Status epilepticus is usually defined as prolonged or recurrent tonic–clonic seizures persisting for 30 minutes or more. However, in clinical practice patients should be aggressively treated if they have more than 5–10 minutes of continuous seizures or two or more discrete seizures between which there is an incomplete recovery of consciousness.

➤ It has been estimated that the incidence of status is 18–28 cases per 100 000 of the population, with a mortality rate of 20%.

➤ Status is more common in children, patients with learning difficulties and those with structural brain lesions. The most common factors precipitating status in patients with an established diagnosis of epilepsy are drug withdrawal, intercurrent illness, metabolic disturbance or progression of the underlying disease.

➤ The following are the general principles of treating status (each hospital should have its own protocol and all staff should be familiar with it):

➤ Maintain the airway, assess the breathing and give oxygen, maintain the circulation, establishing intravenous (IV) access; take blood for emergency investigation (full blood count, glucose, renal and liver function tests, calcium level and AEDs level).

➤ Give dextrose if there is a possibility of hypoglycaemia or thiamine if there is a history of alcohol abuse.

➤ Lorazepam as IV bolus should be given initially (diazepam intravenously or rectally could be used), followed by phenytoin infusion. IV fosphenytoin infusion is an alternative. IV valproate infusion is considered to be as effective. ECG, blood pressure monitoring and pulse oximetry are needed.

- If status continues the patient should be transferred to the intensive care unit and propofol, thiopental or midazolam should be started after discussion with the intensivist. EEG monitoring is needed in anaesthetised patients.
- If the patient is known to have epilepsy the regular AEDs should be given orally or through a nasogastric tube. Maintenance AEDs should be started in patients not known to have seizures.

WOMEN AND EPILEPSY

- A baby with a major congenital malformation such as neural tube defect is the main concern for any woman taking AEDs. If possible, AEDs should be stopped in the planning stages of any pregnancy. However, this is usually difficult in clinical practice, hence the need for a clear explanation of the teratogenic effects of AEDs.
- The background risk of birth defects in the general population is 1%–3%, doubling in patients on monotherapy (6%), and tripling in patients on dual therapy (9%). Polytherapy carries a risk of up to 20%. Sodium valproate can cause foetal valproate syndrome, which has dysmorphic features.
- Any woman on AEDs should take 5 mg of folic acid daily if she is planning pregnancy, as this may reduce the risk of any neural tube defects. Babies born to patients taking enzyme-inducing AEDs should receive 1 mg of vitamin K intramuscularly at birth to reduce the risk of haemorrhagic disease of the newborn.
- Breastfeeding should be encouraged, as the amount of AEDs excreted in the breast milk is too small to cause any significant problems to babies.
- Women on enzyme-inducing AEDs should avoid using a progestogen-only pill or a combined oral contraceptive pill containing less than 50 mcg of oestrogen, as drug interactions can lead to failure of the oral contraceptive pill.

OTHER ASPECTS OF EPILEPSY

➤ The diagnosis of epilepsy can have huge social implications due to the stigma attached. Employers tend to be reluctant to offer jobs to people with epilepsy, which can encourage social isolation.

➤ Patients should be advised about possible dangers they can face from bathing, swimming, cycling and using sharp implements or dangerous machinery.

➤ Alcohol may provoke seizures and should be consumed in moderation. Sleep deprivation could also lower the seizure threshold.

➤ In the UK, patients with seizures are not allowed to drive cars or motorcycles unless they are seizure-free for 1 year, or have had attacks only during sleep for 3 years. For driving large lorries and passenger-carrying vehicles the requirement is 10 years of seizure-freedom without taking AEDs.

➤ Sudden unexpected death in epilepsy (SUDEP) is increasingly recognised as a major cause of death in patients with chronic epilepsy. It is defined as sudden, unexpected, witnessed or unwitnessed, non-traumatic and non-drowning death in patients with epilepsy, with or without evidence of a seizure, and excluding documented status epilepticus, in which post-mortem examination does not reveal a toxicological or anatomic cause for death. The cause of SUDEP is not clear. It is recommended that tailored information and discussion about this issue should be part of the counselling of patients.

CHAPTER 19

Stroke

➤ Stroke is a common neurological disorder, the second most common overall cause of death and a major cause of disability in survivors.

➤ Incidence of stroke is around 250 per 100 000 of the population per year in developed countries. The incidence increases with age.

➤ Stroke is defined by the World Health Organization as 'a clinical syndrome consisting of rapidly developing clinical signs of focal (at times global) disturbance of cerebral function, lasting more than 24 hours or leading to death with no apparent cause other than that of vascular origin'.

➤ Transient ischaemic attack (TIA) is defined as stroke symptoms and signs that resolve within 24 hours. However, in the majority of patients the TIA symptoms usually resolve within minutes or a few hours at most.

➤ A non-disabling stroke is defined as 'a stroke with symptoms that last for more than 24 hours but later resolve, leaving no permanent disability'.

TYPES OF STROKE

➤ Ischaemic: the most common type of stroke (80%). Ischaemic stroke is due to reduction of the blood supply to the brain as a result of occlusion of arteries. The ischaemic stroke could be due to:

➤ Thrombosis – usually as the site of an atheromatous plaque.
➤ Embolism – as a result from ulceration and fragmentation of atheromatous plaque. Less commonly, the heart can be the source of the emboli.
➤ Small-vessel disease – due to atheroma of the small penetrating arteries leading to 'lacunar infarction'.

➤ Haemorrhagic – due to rupture of the arteries, causing either intracerebral or subarachnoid haemorrhage.

CEREBRAL CIRCULATION

➤ The cerebral hemispheres are supplied by:
  ➤ Anterior circulation – formed by the internal carotid arteries and its branches, the middle cerebral arteries and the anterior cerebral arteries.
  ➤ Posterior circulation – formed by the two vertebral arteries that join to form the basilar artery, which bifurcates to two posterior cerebral arteries.
➤ The anterior communicating artery connects the middle cerebral artery and the anterior cerebral artery, while the posterior communicating artery connects the middle cerebral artery and posterior cerebral artery, forming the circle of Willis.
➤ The small (penetrating) vessels are branches from all the aforementioned arteries.
➤ Anterior circulation supplies the frontal, parietal and temporal lobes and the eyes (hence amaurosis fugax) while the posterior circulation supplies occipital lobes, cerebellum, brainstem and the thalamus.

CLINICAL PATTERNS OF ISCHAEMIC STROKE

➤ Anterior circulation ischaemia (carotid territory) is the most common pattern, comprising of around 50% of strokes, and leads to hemiparesis with or without sensory loss, homonymous hemianopia, dysphagia, dysphasia (dominant hemisphere) and dysarthria.

➤ Posterior circulation ischaemia (vertebrobasilar territory) comprises around 25% of strokes and leads to vertigo, diplopia, ataxia, cortical blindness, hemiparesis or tetraparesis.
➤ Features such as hemiparesis, homonymous hemianopia, dysphagia and dysarthria can be due to anterior or posterior circulation ischaemia.
➤ Lacunar strokes comprise 25% of strokes and present with one of the following four patterns:
  ➤ pure motor hemiparesis due to lacunar infarction in internal capsule or pons
  ➤ hemisensorimotor pattern due to lacunar infarction in internal capsule, pons or corona radiata
  ➤ ataxic hemiparesis due to lacunar infarction in internal capsule or pons
  ➤ pure hemisensory pattern due to lacunar infarction in the thalamus.

VASCULAR RISK FACTORS

➤ Hypertension.
➤ Diabetes.
➤ Hyperlipidaemia.
➤ Family history of atheromatous diseases (stroke or ischaemic heart disease).
➤ Smoking.
➤ Previous history of TIA or stroke.
➤ Cardiac diseases associated with embolic stroke, such as atrial fibrillation, mitral valve disease, mural thrombus following myocardial infarction and bacterial endocarditis.

HAEMORRHAGIC STROKE

➤ There are two main types of haemorrhagic stroke:
  ➤ intracerebral haemorrhage
  ➤ subarachnoid haemorrhage.

Intracerebral haemorrhage

➤ Intracerebral haemorrhage usually presents with sudden onset of severe neurological deficit with headache. However, intracerebral haemorrhage cannot be differentiated from ischaemic stroke on clinical grounds. Therefore, a brain CT is essential.

➤ The most common cause of intracerebral haemorrhage is hypertension due to rupture of the small penetrating arteries and typically occurs in the basal ganglia. Other sites of the bleeding are lobar white matter, pons and cerebellum.

➤ Anticoagulants and arteriovenous malformations can cause intracerebral haemorrhage.

Subarachnoid haemorrhage

➤ Patient presents with sudden onset of severe headache associated with vomiting and neck stiffness. The headache peaks within seconds. Patients usually have neurological deficit but may present *only* with acute headache.

➤ The most common cause of subarachnoid haemorrhage is the rupture of intracranial aneurysm on the circle of Willis.

➤ Brain CT is essential in diagnosing subarachnoid haemorrhage. However, the brain CT can be normal. If the brain CT is normal then a LP should be performed around 6–8 hours after the onset of the symptoms, looking for bloodstained CSF (xanthochromia). Spectrophotometry is needed to confirm the xanthochromia.

➤ Subarachnoid haemorrhage can lead to complications such as rebleeding or secondary ischaemia due to vasospasm.

INVESTIGATIONS

➤ Conditions that may mimic stroke, such as brain tumour, subdural haematoma and cerebral abscess, should be excluded by brain scan. Brain CT can be normal in the early stages of ischaemic stroke.

➤ Full blood count, biochemical profile including fasting glucose, ECG and chest X-ray should be considered for all patients with stroke.

➤ If a cardiac source of emboli is suspected, then consider

transthoracic or transoesophageal echocardiography and 24-hour ECG.

➤ If the stroke is in the carotid territory then consider carotid Doppler ultrasound.

➤ Patients with TIA and non-disabling stroke should be investigated along similar lines to stroke patients.

MANAGEMENT OF STROKE

➤ It is important to remember that stroke is a preventable (primary and secondary prevention) and treatable disease.

➤ Ideally all patients with acute stroke should be managed within a 'stroke unit that offers a multidisciplinary and well-organised stroke service'. Involvement of physiotherapists, speech therapists and occupational therapists is essential.

➤ If a patient presents within 4½ hours from the onset of the stroke symptoms an urgent brain CT is needed to exclude cerebral haemorrhage followed by thrombolysis with IV alteplase. The earlier the treatment is given the better the potential outcome for the patient.

➤ Patients presenting outside the thrombolysis window should have a brain CT as soon as possible (not more than 24 hours) to exclude cerebral haemorrhage, followed by 300 mg of aspirin.

➤ Assessment of swallowing is essential before the patient is given any oral fluid, food or medication to prevent aspiration pneumonia.

➤ Early mobilisation of the patient with stroke is essential to prevent complications such as deep-vein thrombosis, bedsores and contractures.

➤ A period of rehabilitation may be needed. Social services involvement may be required.

➤ Secondary prevention includes the following measures:
  ➤ Long-term aspirin. If patient is allergic to or cannot tolerate aspirin, dipyridamole or clopidogrel can be used.
  ➤ Anticoagulation is indicated in patients with atrial fibrillation.

➤ Control blood pressure. A combination of diuretic and angiotensin-converting enzyme inhibitor was found to be useful in preventing stroke, even in patients with normal blood pressure.

➤ Statins, even if patient's serum cholesterol level is normal.

➤ Manage any other modifiable risk factors such as diabetes and smoking.

➤ Patients who make a reasonable recovery and are found to have a significant internal carotid artery stenosis (> 70%) should benefit from carotid endarterectomy.

➤ Measures of secondary prevention also apply in patients with TIA and non-disabling stroke.

➤ Young patients with severe middle cerebral artery infarction may need decompressive hemicraniectomy.

➤ Intracerebral haemorrhage is usually treated conservatively. However, surgical evacuation of the haematoma may be indicated if the neurological status of the patient deteriorates or if the patient develops hydrocephalus. Treating hypertension is the best way to prevent intracerebral haemorrhage.

➤ Once a diagnosis of subarachnoid haemorrhage is confirmed, the patient should be transferred to a neurosurgical unit to determine the source of bleeding by CTA, MRA or cerebral angiogram. Nimodipine and IV fluids should be given to reduce the risk of secondary ischaemia. Surgical clipping or coiling of the aneurysm is the main treatment.

OTHER TYPES OF STROKE

Cerebrovenous sinus thrombosis

➤ Thrombosis in the cerebral venous system is relatively uncommon.

➤ Patients may present with headache, seizure and focal neurological signs. A patient could also present with headache and papilloedema mimicking idiopathic intracranial hypertension.

➤ CVST may be associated with pregnancy and the oral contraceptive pill. Hypercoagulability disorders need to be excluded and therefore a full thrombophilia screen is essential. Otitis media and mastoiditis can cause CVST.

➤ Brain CT can identify venous infarction. CTV or MRV is usually diagnostic, although cerebral angiography with venography may be needed in some cases.

➤ The mainstay of the treatment is anticoagulation.

Dissection of the cervicocerebral arteries

➤ Dissection of internal carotid or vertebral arteries is relatively rare.

➤ Trauma, even trivial, is a well-known cause of dissection.

➤ Headache or neck pain is common. Horner's syndrome is another feature. Dissection usually leads to thromboembolic stroke affecting the carotid or the posterior circulation tertiary.

➤ CTA or MRA is usually diagnostic although cerebral angiography may be needed in some cases.

➤ There is no clear agreement about the best treatment for dissection although aspirin or anticoagulants are often used.

PROGNOSIS

➤ The prognosis depends on the type and the severity of the stroke. However, generally:
  - ➤ 30% die at 1 year and 60% at 5 years
  - ➤ 30% are dependent at 1 year
  - ➤ 30% have a further stroke before 5 years.

CHAPTER 20

Parkinson's disease

➤ Parkinson's disease (PD) is a common progressive neurodegenerative disease that was first described by James Parkinson in 1817.

➤ It is a disease of the basal ganglia (extra-pyramidal). The basal ganglia includes the following nuclei that have a rather complicated interconnection:

➤ putamen
➤ caudate
➤ globus pallidus
➤ substantia nigra.

➤ The combination of bradykinesia (slowness of movement), rigidity (increased resistance to passive extension and flexion), tremor (mainly resting) and postural abnormalities are called Parkinsonism. PD is the most frequent cause of Parkinsonism.

➤ PD has an incidence of around 4–20 per 100 000 of the population per year, and prevalence of 100–180 per 100 000 of the population. The prevalence of the disease increases with age and about 2% of people > 65 years have PD.

➤ The mean age at onset of PD is between 55 and 65 years, with a slight male predominance of 60%.

PATHOLOGY

➤ PD is characterised pathologically by loss of pigment from the substantia nigra with neuronal loss and the presence of Lewy bodies in the surviving neurons.

➤ Lewy bodies are eosinophilic intracytoplasmic inclusions. They are not specific for PD, and are reported in other neurodegenerative disorders.

AETIOLOGY

➤ The exact cause of PD is not known. It is possible that the disease is a result of interaction between several environmental and genetic factors.

➤ Several potential environmental factors were suggested. A viral cause for PD was entertained after patients who survived the 1920s epidemic of von Economo's encephalitis developed Parkinsonism. However, there is no evidence to support infection as an aetiologic factor for PD. MPTP (1-methyl-4-phenyl-1,2,3,6,-tetrahydropyridine) was found to cause severe non-progressive Parkinsonism when it was injected intravenously by a group of drug addicts in the United States. This led to a widespread search for toxins as a cause of PD but no specific toxin was found to cause PD.

➤ PD is a sporadic disease. However, up to 20% of patients have a positive family history with only 1%–2% having the familial form of PD. Both autosomal recessive and dominant forms have been described. Gene mutations implicated in the development of PD have been described.

CLINICAL FEATURES

➤ The onset of disease is usually asymmetrical.

➤ Patients usually present with non-specific aches and pains, stiffness, reduced handwriting size, general slowing down or depression and sleep disturbance.

➤ Tremor is the presenting feature in 70% of patients. Some patients have tremor with minimal bradykinesia or rigidity, hence the name 'benign tremulous Parkinson's disease'.

➤ Examination usually shows loss of arm swing when walking, tendency to drag a leg, difficulty with hand movements, stooped posture and loss of facial expression. Other typical features are reduced voice volume, lead-pipe rigidity or cogwheel rigidity if tremor is superimposed and the pill-rolling resting tremor.

➤ In the late stages of PD patients develop speech and swallowing difficulties. Other features of the late stages of the disease are falls, gait problems, autonomic dysfunction and dementia.

DIFFERENTIAL DIAGNOSIS

Essential tremor

➤ Essential tremor (ET) is the most common movement disorder, with an estimated prevalence of between 4 and 39 per 1000 of the population. The annual incidence is about 23 per 100 000 of the population. Men and women are equally affected.

➤ ET is a familial disorder and around 50% of patients report a positive family history. There are no specific pathological features of ET.

➤ Typically the tremor is postural, occurring while voluntarily maintaining position against gravity. This mainly involves the hands and forearms, starting intermittently and progressing to become permanent, rarely remitting and usually worsened by emotion. Tremor of the head, voice, tongue and legs may follow. There is no rigidity or bradykinesia.

➤ Treatment is mainly with beta blockers – particularly propranolol. Primidone can have a beneficial effect but the majority of patients do not tolerate it. Up to 60% of ET patients report an improvement in their tremor after consuming alcohol.

Vascular Parkinsonism

➤ Common in older patients with a history of hypertension, who usually present with gait difficulty, symmetrical rigidity, absent tremor and no or some response to levodopa therapy.

➤ There are no generally accepted clinical criteria to diagnose vascular Parkinsonism. There is also no specific treatment but a trial of levodopa is worth considering.

Drug-induced Parkinsonism

➤ Drug-induced Parkinsonism can occur with neuroleptics such as phenothiazines and butyrophenones. This occurs in 10%–15% of psychotic patients treated with these drugs.

➤ Antiemetic drugs such as prochlorperazine and metoclopramide can cause Parkinsonism. Other drugs such as sodium valproate, tetrabenazine and calcium-channel blockers such as cinnarizine are also reported to cause Parkinsonism.

➤ Stopping the offending drug is obviously the treatment of choice in drug-induced Parkinsonism. However, this can be difficult, especially with neuroleptic drugs.

➤ Anticholinergics and amantadine may help to reduce the Parkinsonian symptoms in patients with drug-induced Parkinsonism.

Parkinson's plus syndromes

➤ They are a group of neurodegenerative disorders that share some features with PD but have different pathological features and do not respond to dopaminergic therapy.

➤ Progressive supranuclear palsy where there is postural instability and falls, symmetrical bradykinesia and rigidity, cognitive impairment, dysarthria and speech changes and vertical downgaze palsy.

➤ Multiple system atrophy where there is symmetrical bradykinesia and rigidity features of autonomic dysfunction and cerebellar and pyramidal signs.

Wilson's disease

➤ Wilson's disease is a rare but treatable disease; therefore, it should not be missed. It is an autosomal recessive disorder due to impairment in the copper transport system and deficiency of the copper-carrying plasma protein caeruloplasmin, leading to copper deposition in all the body's tissue.

➤ PD rarely affects young people; therefore, any patient below the age of 40 presenting with Parkinsonism should be screened for Wilson's disease.

➤ Serum caeruloplasmin is almost always low, which is associated with low serum copper and high urinary copper excretion.

➤ Kayser–Fleischer rings (deposition of copper in Descemet's membrane of the cornea which will appear brown or grey) are present in all patients with neurological features of Wilson's disease, so slit lamp examination is essential.

➤ Several medications can be used in treating Wilson's disease. Chelating agents, such as penicillamine, are effective treatments. Other medications such as zinc sulfate or acetate can be used.

MANAGEMENT

➤ PD is a chronic progressive disease and establishing a good relationship between the patient and the treating physician is essential. Patients should be realistically informed about the prognosis and expectation from treatment. Every effort should be made to support patients throughout the course of the disease. Patient-oriented leaflets, booklets and websites help patients to understand the nature of their disease.

➤ Dopamine agonists are widely used as the first choice, in the hope of reducing the long-term motor complications of levodopa, especially in younger patients.

➤ There is no drug that is proven to slow the progress of the disease.

Dopamine agonists

➤ Dopamine agonists act directly on the postsynaptic dopamine receptors. Drug-induced motor complications are less frequent and less severe than levodopa. Therefore, dopamine agonists have been advocated as the drugs that delay the introduction of levodopa. They are used as monotherapy or adjuvant therapy.

➤ Some patients experience dizziness, hypotensive reactions, nausea and vomiting initially. Adding domperidone during the initiation phase can counteract this.

➤ Currently non-ergot derivative dopamine agonists such as pramipexole, ropinirole, rotigotine (self-adhesive patches) and apomorphine are used.

➤ Apomorphine hydrochloride is indicated in patients with refractory motor fluctuations. It can only be given as a subcutaneous injection or continuous subcutaneous infusion.

Levodopa

➤ Levodopa was introduced in the late 1960s and is still the most effective drug treatment in PD – 'the gold standard therapy'. It is metabolised to dopamine by aromatic L-amino acid decarboxylase and is then stored in and released by the nigrostriatal neurons. Levodopa is always given with a peripheral decarboxylase inhibitor, either carbidopa or benserazide, to prevent peripheral dopamine formation and to reduce side effects such as nausea and vomiting.

➤ Almost every patient with PD responds to levodopa therapy. Initially patients respond very well to levodopa – the 'honeymoon period'; however, after around 3–5 years of treatment, levodopa-related motor complications usually emerge:

  ➤ Wearing-off – the beneficial effect of levodopa wears off quickly and patients may need more frequent doses.
  ➤ On–off phenomena – patient's condition fluctuates from good treatment effect ('on') to severe Parkinsonian state ('off') with no relation to levodopa dosing regime.
  ➤ Dyskinesia – drug-induced purposeless involuntary movements that affect upper or lower limbs, as well as the neck and trunk.

➤ These levodopa-related motor complications can be mild and cause no major disability. However, as the disease progresses, they become more troublesome and difficult to manage.

➤ Duodopa, which is levodopa as a concentrated intestinal gel, can be used in patients with refractory motor fluctuations. However, it requires insertion of a percutaneous gastrostomy tube.

Catechol-O-methyl transferase inhibitors

➤ Levodopa is metabolised by catechol-O-methyl transferase (COMT) to inactive products both in the peripheral blood and in the brain. COMT inhibitors increase the amount of dopamine available by reducing the metabolism of levodopa. They are used to reduce wearing-off effects. Nausea, vomiting, abdominal pain, constipation and diarrhoea are possible side effects with COMT inhibitors.

➤ Entacapone is widely used and a single preparation combining levodopa, carbidopa (peripheral decarboxylase inhibitor) and entacapone is available (Stalevo).

Monoamine oxidase B inhibitors

➤ Intracerebral monoamine oxidase B (MAOB) metabolises dopamine. Blocking this process increases the amount of endogenous dopamine. Selegiline and rasagiline are used both as monotherapy and as adjuvant treatment. MAOB inhibitors can cause constipation, nausea, postural hypotension and hallucinations as side effects.

Anticholinergics

➤ Anticholinergics such as trihexyphenidyl hydrochloride and orphenadrine hydrochloride can help in treating tremor. However, they may cause dry mouth, confusion, hallucinations and urinary retention, especially in older patients, and therefore they are of limited use.

Amantadine

➤ As an antiviral agent amantadine was also found by chance to improve the symptoms of PD. It is an N-methyl-D-aspartate receptor antagonist and not widely used nowadays except to treat dyskinesia. As it may cause confusion and hallucinations, it is better not to use it in patients with neuropsychiatric symptoms.

Surgical treatment

➤ Bilateral subthalamic nucleus stimulation has replaced pallidotomy as the operation of choice in patients with PD. It is indicated in patients with motor complications not responding to medical treatment. The patients have to be responsive to levodopa with no significant neuropsychiatric problems or active comorbidity.

Treating the non-motor symptoms

➤ Depression is common and should be treated with antidepressants such as selective serotonin reuptake inhibitors. Hallucinations and psychosis can be difficult to manage and are best treated with atypical antipsychotics. There is some evidence that cholinesterase inhibitors may help PD dementia. Physiotherapy, occupational therapy and speech therapy can be of help to some patients especially if they experience falls.

PROGNOSIS

➤ The effect of PD on survival is not clear; however, the disease has a greater effect on younger patients because of their longer life expectancy.
➤ Tremor-dominant patients have a better prognosis than those without tremor (akinetic-rigid presentation).
➤ Patients with end-stage PD usually die from infections such as bronchopneumonia.

CHAPTER 21

Multiple sclerosis

➤ MS is a chronic inflammatory demyelinating disease of the brain and spinal cord (CNS), and one of the commonest disabling neurological diseases among young people in developed countries.

➤ MS affects 1 in 800–1000 people in the UK.

➤ MS usually presents in patients aged 20–40 years.

PATHOLOGY

➤ MS is characterised pathologically by loss of myelin (inflammatory process) with possible secondary axonal damage (degenerative process).

➤ The hallmark of MS is white-matter lesions affecting the CNS, commonly in the periventricular areas, corpus callosum, optic nerve, brainstem, cerebellum and cervical spine.

➤ The immune system is involved in MS pathogenesis, although its exact role is not clear.

AETIOLOGY

➤ The exact cause of MS is not known. It is possible that the disease is a result of interaction between several environmental and genetic factors.

➤ There are geographical and latitudinal effects on the prevalence of MS; increased distance from the equator increases the prevalence of the disease. Also, migration from a high- to a low-risk area before the age of 15 reduces the MS risk and vice versa.

➤ There is an association between MS and Human Leukocyte antigen types.

➤ There is increased incidence of MS in those with an affected first-degree relative.

CLINICAL FEATURES

Optic neuritis

➤ Common presentation of MS.

➤ Pain worse on moving the eyes and visual impairment (varying from mild to severe) are the typical symptoms of optic neuritis.

➤ There are two types of optic neuritis:

   ➤ *Retrobulbar (posterior)* – common form of optic neuritis. The optic disc appears normal.

   ➤ *Papillitis (anterior)* – less common form of optic neuritis. The optic disc is usually red and swollen with exudate and haemorrhages.

➤ Examination shows reduced visual acuity, central scotoma, loss of colour vision and relative afferent pupillary defect (*see* p. 35).

➤ Complete or near complete visual recovery over a period of weeks or months is the usual outcome.

Sensory and motor features

➤ Sensory symptoms such as numbness and pins and needles are common and can affect any part of the body.

➤ Weakness affects the lower limbs more commonly than the upper limbs. The motor deficit is of UMN type and usually leads to spastic paraplegia.

Brainstem and cerebellum

➤ Dizziness and vertigo.

➤ Double vision usually due to a lesion in the pathways that maintain conjugate eye movement rather than a specific cranial nerve abnormality.

➤ Internuclear ophthalmoplegia: when patient looks to the right or left, there is ataxic nystagmus in the abducted eye and failure to adduct the other eye, due to a lesion in the medial longitudinal fasciculus. This connects the 3rd nerve nuclus on one side with the 6th nerve nucleus on the other side.

➤ Limb or gait ataxia.

➤ Dysarthria.

Other features

➤ Fatigue is common.

➤ Bladder and bowel dysfunction.

➤ Sexual problems.

➤ Depression, euphoria and cognitive impairment.

TYPES OF MS

➤ Relapsing–remitting MS (the most common presentation): neurological episodes with variable recovery but with stability in between the episodes.

➤ Relapsing–remitting with secondary progressive MS: neurological episodes superimposed on a progressive course. This usually begins as relapsing–remitting disease.

➤ Primary progressive MS: gradual development of neurological deficits from the onset without any relapses.

DIAGNOSIS

➤ MS is a clinical diagnosis but brain MRI and CSF analysis are important.

➤ The occurrence of the lesions in CNS (clinically and radiologically), which are disseminated in time and place (at least two separate episodes).

➤ Brain MRI is abnormal in 95% of patients with MS. The multiple white-matter lesions are characteristically seen in periventricular areas, corpus callosum, brainstem and cerebellum. Active lesions are enhanced with gadolinium.

➤ Routine CSF analysis is usually normal. Oligoclonal bands that are positive in CSF but not in the blood are found in 95% of patients with MS and indicate intrathecal immunoglobulin synthesis.

➤ Remember that multiple white-matter lesions in brain MRI are also seen in other disorders such as cerebral ischaemia, neurosarcoid and vasculitis. Also, oligoclonal bands in CSF are positive in other inflammatory conditions such as autoimmune disorders and neurosarcoid.

➤ Visual evoked responses (a neurophysiological study) can be delayed in patients with MS. However, they are not widely used.

MANAGEMENT

➤ Explaining to newly diagnosed patients the nature of MS is vital, emphasising that the disease can follow a benign course. Severe disability (becoming wheelchair bound) is a possibility but not a certainty.

➤ Always encourage the patient to live a normal life.

Symptomatic treatment

➤ Baclofen and tizanidine are used to treat spasticity.

➤ Fatigue is difficult to treat. Fluoxetine, amantadine and modafinil are used with very limited success.

➤ Pain is common and should be treated with amitriptyline or gabapentin.

➤ Depression is treated with the usual antidepressants.

➤ A full urinary bladder assessment may be needed by a urologist. Anticholinergic drugs such as oxybutynin help with the bladder instability. Laxatives help in constipation. Patients with sexual problems will need help from a sexual dysfunction clinic.

Treating the relapses

➤ IV methylprednisolone (1 g daily for 3 days) is commonly used to shorten the duration of relapse without any influence on the long-term outcome. Although it can be used in patients with progressive disease, the response is usually limited.

➤ A short course of rehabilitation is useful, especially after a relapse.

Disease-modifying treatments

➤ Disease-modifying treatments such as beta interferons and glatiramer acetate have been shown to reduce the number of relapses by one-third. In the UK the disease-modifying treatments are usually given to patients with relapsing–remitting disease who fulfill the following criteria:
  ➢ aged 18 or older
  ➢ can walk for at least 100 metres without assistance
  ➢ have had at least two relapses in the past 2 years.

PROGNOSIS

➤ The prognosis is variable. Poor prognostic indicators include male gender, high number of relapses, motor or cerebellar presentations and progressive course.
➤ Probably one-third of patients have a mild form of MS. However, life expectancy is reduced by 5–10 years and there is a 50% chance of a patient losing their ability to walk independently after 15 years.

OTHER DEMYELINATING DISEASES

Neuromyelitis optica (Devic's disease)

➤ A monophasic disease consisting of a combination of optic neuritis and myelitis (inflammation of the spinal cord) occurring simultaneously or in succession.
➤ Brain MRI is normal while the spinal MRI shows demyelination lesions extending over three or more vertebral segments. Oligoclonal bands are usually negative in the CSF. Aquaporin antibodies can be detected in the patient's serum.
➤ The disease is usually aggressive and patients are left with severe disabilities. IV methylprednisolone, IV immunoglobulin and immunosuppressive agents are used to treat NMO.

Acute disseminated encephalomyelitis

➤ Acute disseminated encephalomyelitis (ADEM) is a monophasic fulminant demyelinating syndrome, more common in children (after immunisation).

➤ ADEM usually presents with encephalopathy (seizures, meningism) and features of myelitis, cerebral or cerebellar involvement. Half of the patients affected report a preceding infectious illness.

➤ Brain and spinal MRI show demyelination lesions, and oligoclonal bands are positive in the CSF in around one-third of the patients.

➤ The disease is treated with IV methylprednisolone and/or IV immunoglobulin.

PART IV

Neurological problems and diseases – others

CHAPTER 22

Infections of the central nervous system

➤ Meningitis is inflammation of the meninges; encephalitis is inflammation of the brain.
➤ Different bacteria and viruses can cause acute meningitis, and certain viruses can lead to encephalitis. However, there is always a degree of overlap between the meningitis and encephalitis (meningoencephalitis). The infective process can involve a local area of the brain (cerebritis) leading to cerebral abscess.

AETIOLOGY

➤ Acute bacterial meningitis is usually caused by:
  ➤ streptococcus pneumoniae
  ➤ neisseria meningitidis
  ➤ haemophilus influenzae.
➤ The most common cause of viral meningitis is enteroviruses.
➤ Herpes simplex virus is a well-recognised cause of encephalitis.
➤ Cerebral abscess is usually a result of:
  ➤ spread of local infection such as sinuses or middle ear infection
  ➤ traumatic head injury

➤ haematological dissemination such as that seen in bronchiectasis

➤ immunocompromised patients.

CLINICAL FEATURES

➤ Non-specific features such as fever and rigors.

➤ Features related to meningeal irritation such as headache, photophobia and neck stiffness (positive Kernig's sign).

➤ Features of raised intracranial pressure such as headache, vomiting, impairment of consciousness and papilloedema.

➤ Encephalitic features such as focal neurological deficit, seizures and impairment of consciousness.

➤ Cerebral abscess tends to present with fever, headache, focal neurological deficit and seizures.

➤ Viral meningitis is a benign disease and presents with headache and fever with no impairment of consciousness.

➤ Meningococcal purpuric rash may be seen with meningococcal meningitis.

INVESTIGATIONS

➤ Full blood count may show high white cell count.

➤ High ESR or C-reactive protein.

➤ Blood cultures could help to identify the organism in bacterial infection.

➤ Brain CT is normal in meningitis. Brain MRI may show temporal lobe changes in herpes simplex encephalitis. A ring-enhancing lesion with surrounding oedema points to a cerebral abscess.

➤ CSF analysis is vital to confirm the diagnosis and to identify the organism (brain CT is easily available in all acute hospitals and therefore it must be done before LP in any patients with suspected neurological infections). Bacterial meningitis leads to high white cell counts in the CSF (> 200/mm^3) mainly polymorphs with high protein and low glucose. Viral meningitis, on the other hand, causes raised white cell counts in the CSF (< 200/mm^3) mainly lymphocytes with slightly raised protein and normal glucose. Partially treated bacterial meningitis could alter the CSF analysis. Herpes simplex encephalitis leads to high white cell counts in the CSF (up to 500/mm^3) mainly lymphocytes with slightly raised protein and normal glucose. Polymerase chain reaction (PCR) for herpes virus in CSF is positive in the majority of the patients with herpes simplex encephalitis. LP is not indicated in cerebral abscesses.

MANAGEMENT

➤ IV treatment with a broad-spectrum antibiotic (third-generation cephalosporin such as ceftriaxone) and acyclovir should be started immediately and continued until the diagnosis is clear. The antibiotic could be altered once the organism and the sensitivities are identified.

➤ IV dexamethasone for a period of 4 days was found to be effective in reducing unfavourable outcome in acute bacterial meningitis. The first dose of dexamethasone should be given with the first dose of antibiotic.

➤ Antimicrobial treatment and surgical intervention are needed to treat cerebral abscesses.

➤ No specific treatment is needed for viral meningitis, as it is a self-limiting disease.

➤ Acute complications such as hydrocephalus should be treated.

➤ Patients with acute CNS infections may need intensive supportive measures in high-dependence or intensive care units.

PROGNOSIS

➤ Acute CNS infections still carry a high mortality rate (around 20%), especially if there is a delay in starting treatment.

➤ Patients may have long-term sequelae such as epilepsy and cognitive impairments.

OTHER INFECTIONS OF THE NERVOUS SYSTEM

Tuberculous meningitis

➤ Asian, immigrant and immunocompromised patients are at a higher risk of catching tuberculous meningitis (TBM).

➤ The onset is usually subacute and patients could have non-specific symptoms such as headaches, fever and weight loss. Patients may develop seizures and cranial nerve abnormalities.

➤ CSF is vital in making the diagnosis. There is usually high protein (> 1.0 g/L), lymphocytes (50–500/mm³) and low glucose (< 50% of the blood glucose). Ziehl–Neelsen stain is usually negative and cultures are positive in 60% of cases; it normally takes several weeks to obtain the results.

➤ Brain CT and/or MRI may show basal meningeal enhancement. Hydrocephalus, ischaemic infarction or tuberculomas (slow-growing granulomas) can be seen. Chest X-ray may show evidence of pulmonary tuberculosis.

➤ Treatment with antituberculous drugs should be started as soon as possible. Dexamethasone is widely used.

Cryptococcal meningitis

➤ Fungal infection usually seen in immunocompromised patients.

➤ Cryptococcal meningitis may present with non-specific headache, fever and cranial nerve palsies and seizures resembling TBM.

➤ Brain CT and/or MRI may show mass lesions (cryptococcomas).

➤ CSF shows high protein, lymphocytosis and low glucose. A CSF India ink preparation is positive in 50% of cases.

➤ Antifungal therapy such as fluconazole or amphotericin B should be started as soon as possible.

CHAPTER 23

Guillain–Barré syndrome

➤ GBS is the most common cause of acute flaccid paralysis in the Western world.
➤ GBS has an annual incidence of 2–4 per 100 000 of the population.

CLINICAL FEATURES
➤ Patients present with rapid progressive ascending paralysis with sensory symptoms (over a week or two).
➤ GBS is predominantly a motor peripheral neuropathy.
➤ The neurological examination shows generalised weakness (tetraparesis) more marked distally with absent reflexes and minimal sensory signs.
➤ Facial weakness (LMN lesion of 7th nerve) and bulbar involvement is common.
➤ There is usually a history of antecedent upper respiratory tract infection or diarrhoea.

INVESTIGATIONS
➤ NCS and/or EMG: important to confirm the diagnosis and usually shows evidence of demyelinating neuropathy.
➤ CSF analysis shows high protein.

MANAGEMENT

➤ IV immunoglobulin is the treatment of choice.
➤ Regular monitoring of forced vital capacity as patients are at risk of respiratory failure.
➤ Regular monitoring of blood pressure and heart rhythm as patients are at risk of autonomic neuropathy.
➤ Low-dose subcutaneous heparin to prevent venous thromboembolism.
➤ Intensive care support as ventilation may be needed.
➤ Neurorehabilitation.

PROGNOSIS

➤ Around 80% of patients make a complete recovery after 1 year. About 5% die and 15% of patients are still unable to walk unaided after 1 year.

CHAPTER 24

Myasthenia gravis

➤ MG is an uncommon autoimmune disorder affecting the neuromuscular junction.
➤ MG has an annual incidence of around 3 per million and a prevalence of 1 in 10 000 of the population.
➤ MG has a bimodal age of onset: 20–40 years of age (predominantly females) and 50–70 years of age (predominantly males).
➤ Patients with MG and their family members have an increased incidence of other autoimmune diseases such as Graves's disease, pernicious anaemia and rheumatoid arthritis.

PATHOPHYSIOLOGY

➤ Acetylcholine is the transmitter at the neuromuscular junction.
➤ In normal circumstances acetylcholine is released from the axon of the LMN to the synape. Acetylcholine then binds to the postsynaptic receptors on the muscle membrane.
➤ In MG autoantibodies (acetylcholine receptor antibodies) block the postsynaptic receptors causing impairment in the neuromuscular transmission.
➤ It is believed that the thymus plays a part in the pathogenesis of MG, but the precise role is not clear.

CLINICAL FEATURES

➤ Ocular symptoms: double vision and/or ptosis.
➤ Speech and swallowing difficulties (bulbar symptoms).
➤ Facial and neck muscle weakness.
➤ Painless limb weakness (mainly proximal muscles), is a common feature of generalised MG (e.g. patient has difficulty lifting the arms above shoulder level).
➤ Respiratory muscles can be affected, leading to breathing difficulties.
➤ Fatigability is very suggestive of MG. The more a muscle is used the weaker it gets. Therefore, symptoms tend to be worse in the evening and after repeated use of the muscle (e.g. difficulty in swallowing is worse at the end of the meal). In the clinic fatigability can be demonstrated by asking the patient to look up for 30–60 seconds. You can see the ptosis get worse. Also, examine shoulder abduction before and after asking the patient to repeatedly abduct the shoulder 20 times. The patient's speech also gets worse as the medical consultation progresses.
➤ Distal limb muscles weakness is rare in MG.
➤ Patients who carry on having only ocular features for 2 years without developing generalised symptoms rarely progress to generalised MG.

INVESTIGATIONS

➤ Acetylcholine receptor antibody is positive in around 90% of patients with generalised MG and 50% of patients with ocular myasthensia. The detection of this antibody is diagnostic of MG. The titre does not correlate with disease severity.
➤ EMG: may show decrement on repetitive stimulation.
➤ Edrophonium (Tensilon) test: rarely used nowadays. It involves injecting a short-acting acetylcholinesterase inhibitor (edrophonium) intravenously, leading to striking improvement of patient's weakness (e.g. ptosis) for 3–5 minutes. However, it can also cause bradycardia, which is reversible with atropine.
➤ Once the diagnosis is confirmed a CT or MRI scan of the thorax is needed to look for thymic hyperplasia or thymoma.

MANAGEMENT

➤ Symptomatic therapy: acetylcholinesterase inhibitors (pyridostigmine) improve the patient's symptoms by slowing the breakdown of acetylcholine, thus increasing its availability in the neuromuscular junction. Side effects such as abdominal cramps and diarrhoea are common and they can be overcome by giving antimuscarinic drugs, such as propantheline.

➤ Immune therapy aiming to suppress the production of the abnormal antibodies. Prednisolone is commonly used. The patient's condition may deteriorate initially (steroid dip), therefore close monitoring is needed. Patients frequently require hospital admission to introduce the prednisolone, especially if patients have bulbar symptoms. Azathioprine is used as a steroid-sparing agent but may take between 6–18 months to work. Patients with severe disease, acutely ill or not responding to oral therapy should be treated with IV immunoglobulin or plasmapheresis.

➤ Patients who are acutely ill with respiratory muscle weakness need close monitoring in hospital by measuring forced vital capacity. Ventilatory support may be needed in patients with forced vital capacity of < 1.5 L.

➤ Thymectomy is indicated in patients with thymoma. Also, it should be considered in young patients (aged < 45 years) with generalised MG.

➤ Some drugs such as aminoglycosides, quinidine, antiarrhythmic drugs, magnesium and benzodiazepines can worsen MG and should be avoided. D-penicillamine can cause MG.

PROGNOSIS

➤ With modern treatment the majority of patients with MG do well and lead a normal life but may need long-term treatment.

➤ The mortality rate is around 4%.

➤ Long-term and spontaneous remission is well recognised but later exacerbation is possible.

CHAPTER 25

Motor neurone disease

➤ MND is a progressive degenerative disease of the motor neurons of the brain, brainstem or spinal cord.
➤ MND has an annual incidence of 1–2 per 100 000 of the population. The median age of onset is 60 years.
➤ MND is a sporadic disease of unknown aetiology. However, 5%–10% of cases are familial.

CLINICAL FEATURES

➤ There are three forms of MND:
  ➤ *Amyotrophic lateral sclerosis* – the most common form. Patient presents with weakness, mainly at hands, with a combination of UMN signs (brisk reflexes) and LMN signs (wasted muscles and fasciculation). The weakness and wasting progresses to other muscles in the trunk and lower limbs.
  ➤ *Progressive bulbar palsy* – patient presents with progressive dysarthria followed by swallowing difficulty. There is wasting and fasciculation of the tongue.
  ➤ *Progressive muscular atrophy* – patient presents with progressive weakness of LMN type.
➤ The majority of patients will have a combination of amyotrophic lateral sclerosis and progressive bulbar palsy.
➤ There are *no* sensory signs or bladder involvement.

➤ Patients die from respiratory failure due to weakness in respiratory muscles and the bulbar palsy.

INVESTIGATIONS

➤ NCS and/or EMG: shows denervation and fasciculations in both wasted and normal muscles.

MANAGEMENT

➤ Multidisciplinary care is needed to provide full support to patients and their carers.
➤ Riluzole, a glutamate antagonist, is widely used as disease-modifying treatment. It may increase survival by a few months.
➤ Percutaneous endoscopic gastrostomy and non-invasive ventilation may be needed.

PROGNOSIS

➤ MND is a relentlessly progressive disease with a survival rate of 3 years.

CHAPTER 26

Dementia

➤ Dementia is a progressive decline in any of the cognitive domains such as memory, language, perception and executive function.
➤ Dementia is becoming a major public health challenge due to the ageing population in both the developed and the developing world. Dementia affects 1% of the population at 60 years of age and 40% of those > 85 years.
➤ The following are risk factors for dementia:
  ➢ age
  ➢ female gender
  ➢ head trauma
  ➢ low level of education
  ➢ vascular risk factors (hypertension, smoking, diabetes)
  ➢ apolipoprotein E.

CLINICAL FEATURES
➤ Patients present with gradual onset of progressive loss of memory and their increased inability to lead a normal life. Patients start to lose their independence and have to rely on spouses and family.
➤ Patients progressively lose their ability to have a normal conversation and they exhibit poor judgement.

➤ Usually patients have no insight into their problems. Also, they may show inappropriate behaviour.

➤ Seizures, especially in the advanced stages of dementia.

CAUSES OF DEMENTIA

Alzheimer's disease

➤ Alzheimer's disease (AD) is the most common cause of dementia (50%–70% of all dementia cases).

➤ AD affects around 5% of the population > 65 years.

➤ AD is a sporadic disease. However, 5%–15% of cases are familial (autosomal dominant affecting younger people) and are associated with gene mutations (amyloid precursor protein gene on chromosome 21, presenilin 1 gene on chromosome 14 and presenilin 2 gene on chromosome 1).

➤ Pathologically there are neurofibrillary tangles and senile plaques, which consist of amyloid-beta protein. Atrophy usually affects temporal lobes.

Dementia with Lewy bodies

➤ Dementia with Lewy bodies causes around 15%–20% of all dementia.

➤ Pathologically there are Lewy bodies (*see* p. 83) both cortically and subcortically.

➤ Patient's usually present with visual hallucinations, fluctuating cognitive impairment and Parkinsonism.

Frontotemporal dementia

➤ Frontotemporal dementia causes around 10% of all dementia.

➤ It usually affects younger patients (< 65 years) and progresses rapidly.

➤ Atrophy affects frontal and temporal lobes.

Vascular dementia

➤ Vascular dementia may result from either small vessel ischaemia leading to diffuse subcortical white matter changes or as a result of multiple recurrent discrete infarcts.

➤ On top of memory problems, patients may develop gait difficulties (*see* pp. 27 and 84) or focal neurology deficits due to specific infarct.

Other causes of dementia

➤ Dementia could be part of other degenerative diseases such as PD and Huntington's disease (HD).
➤ Infectious diseases such as syphilis and HIV/AIDS may cause dementia.
➤ Depression can cause pseudodementia; however, patients with early dementia can develop depression. There is nothing to lose by giving the patient a trial of antidepressants.
➤ Creutzfeldt–Jakob disease (CJD) is very rare and causes rapid progressive dementia (patients usually die within 6 months) with myoclonus and a specific EEG pattern. A new variant of CJD affects younger people and usually presents with psychiatric symptoms and non-specific sensory symptoms. The majority of the new variant of CJD cases have been reported in the UK.

INVESTIGATIONS

➤ The mini-mental state examination (*see* p. 9) is useful as an initial screening tool. However, a full psychometry is more useful to demonstrate all deficits.
➤ Exclude any treatable or modifiable cause of dementia (very rare):
  ➢ brain CT or MRI (hydrocephalus, subdural haematoma, also may show vascular changes)
  ➢ vitamin B_{12}
  ➢ thyroid function test
  ➢ syphilis serology
  ➢ HIV serology.

MANAGEMENT

➤ Multidisciplinary care is needed to provide full support to the patients and their carers.

➤ Full explanation of the diagnosis to the patients and their families is vital.
➤ Treat vascular risk factors in all patients with dementia, not only those with vascular dementia.
➤ Acetylcholinesterase-inhibiting drugs such as donepezil are widely used, especially in AD.
➤ Behavioural and psychiatric problems may need drug treatment – for example, risperidone or quetiapine.

PROGNOSIS
➤ Dementia is a progressive disease and patients usually survive for some years; for example, in AD the survival rate is about 8 years.
➤ The prognosis is worse in older patients, those with the early onset of psychosis and patients with vascular risk factors.

CHAPTER 27

Intracranial tumours

➤ Primary brain tumours are uncommon in comparison with other tumours such as breast and lung cancer.
➤ CNS tumours have an annual incidence of around 6 per 100 000 of the population. The median age of onset is 56 years.

TYPE OF BRAIN TUMOURS

➤ Meningiomas: benign tumours that arise from any part of the meninges.
➤ Gliomas: can be benign or malignant. Histologically they are graded from I to IV, with I being benign and IV being very malignant (glioblastoma multiforme). However, grade I gliomas may progress to become malignant over time.
➤ Metastases: usually from lung or breast cancer.
➤ Pituitary adenomas: the most common is prolactinoma.
➤ Acoustic neuromas: also known as acoustic nerve schwannomas. They are benign tumours arising from the 8th cranial nerve at the cerebellopontine angle.

CLINICAL FEATURES

➤ Features of raised intracranial pressure such as headache, vomiting, papilloedema and false localising sign (6th nerve palsy).

➤ Seizures that can be focal or generalised.
➤ Progressive focal neurological deficit such as hemiplegia and speech impairment. The nature of the deficit depends on the site of the tumour.
➤ Pituitary adenomas may present with visual field defect, usually bitemporal hemianopia and/or endocrine disturbance.
➤ Acoustic neuromas usually present with deafness with 5th and 7th nerve impairment.

INVESTIGATIONS
➤ The investigation of choice to detect brain tumours is brain CT and/or MRI.
➤ If the scans suggest that the tumour can be due to metastatic disease, then searching for the primary tumour is necessary.

MANAGEMENT
➤ Multidisciplinary care is needed to provide full support to the patients and their carers.
➤ Dexamethasone is used to reduce the brain oedema and can help to relieve some of the acute symptoms such as headache. Anticonvulsants are important if the patient is having recurrent seizures.
➤ Partial or complete removal of the tumour is needed in most cases to help in the histological diagnosis. If the tumour is in a part of the brain where an attempt at even partial removal is dangerous, a biopsy may be needed.
➤ Sometimes the tumour is small or inaccessible and repeated brain scans at 3- or 6-month intervals are needed.
➤ Depending on the nature of the tumour, radiotherapy and/or chemotherapy may be necessary.
➤ Prolactinomas respond well to dopamine agonists such as cabergoline.

PROGNOSIS

➤ Benign tumours such as meningiomas, pituitary adenomas and acoustic neuromas carry a very good prognosis although the patient may end up with a residual deficit.

➤ Patients with a low-grade glioma usually survive for many years. However, the progress of a low-grade glioma to a high-grade glioma is common.

➤ Metastases and high-grade gliomas have a poor prognosis.

CHAPTER 28

Head injury

➤ Head injury leading to traumatic brain injury is the most common cause of death and disability in young people in Western countries.
➤ Head injury is more common in men, with a male : female ratio of 2.5 : 1.
➤ In the UK around one million patients present to hospital per year following head injury. The majority (90%) have minor or mild head injuries.

CAUSES OF HEAD INJURY
➤ Road traffic accidents are the main cause of serious head injury.
➤ Falls cause around 40% of head injuries in the UK.
➤ Assaults cause around 20% of head injuries in the UK.
➤ Accidents in the workplace, including sports-related injuries.
➤ Alcohol is a major contributory factor to head injuries.

CLASSIFICATION
➤ Mild head injury: initial score of 13–14 on GCS with no evidence of intracranial pathology. If the GCS score is 15, the head injury can be classified as minor.
➤ Moderate head injury: initial GCS score of 9–12.
➤ Severe head injury: initial GCS score of 3–8.

SHORT-TERM SEQUELA OF HEAD INJURY

➤ Diffuse brain damage:
  ➣ Mild head injury can lead to minimal diffuse damage of the brain.
  ➣ Moderate-to-severe head injury causes diffuse cerebral damage leading to generalised cerebral oedema, which can be severe enough to cause tentorial herniation and coning.
➤ Cerebral haemorrhage such as:
  ➣ intracerebral bleeding
  ➣ subarachnoid haemorrhage
  ➣ acute or chronic subdural haematoma
  ➣ extradural haematoma.
➤ Hypotension and hypoxia, as a result of the head injury or associated body injuries, can lead to ischaemic and hypoxic brain damage.
➤ Skull fractures, which can be simple or depressed. Basal skull fractures can cause CSF rhinorrhoea (CSF leaking through the nose).
➤ CNS infection as a result of open wounds and skull fractures, especially with basal skull fractures.
➤ Seizures, which may aggravate the cerebral hypoxia.

MANAGEMENT

➤ In the UK around 20% of patients with a head injury require admission for observation and less than 5% are managed in neurosurgical units.
➤ All patients with head injuries need initial neurological assessment, which should include GCS, pupil size and any evidence of focal neurological signs. Depending on the severity of the head injury, patients will require neurological observation at regular intervals.
➤ Patients with minor or mild head injury can be discharged after a short period of observation with clear written instructions to return to hospital if they show any signs of deterioration. However, if the patient has any associated medical or social problems hospital admission may be needed.

➤ Patients with moderate-to-severe head injuries need resuscitation ideally in a pre-hospital setting (site of the accident). This includes ABC (maintain clear airway, assess breathing, support the circulation by monitoring the blood pressure, pulse and establish IV line).

➤ Patients with an altered level of consciousness, focal neurological deficit, suspected skull fracture, vomiting or any associated medical problems (on warfarin) will require brain CT.

➤ The management of patients with moderate-to-severe injury should aim to prevent secondary brain damage as a result of hypoxia, hypotension, infection, cerebral haematoma and increased intracranial pressure. Patients may need transferring to a neurosurgical unit, for evacuation of intracranial haematomas, or to intensive care (ideally neurointensive care).

➤ Patients who recovery from moderate-to-severe injury will need a period of neurorehabilitation.

LONG-TERM SEQUELA OF HEAD INJURY

➤ Post-traumatic syndrome: common after a minor, mild head injury. Patients experience non-specific symptoms such as headache, dizziness, lack of concentration, memory problems and poor sleep. Symptoms usually resolve within 12 months. It is not clear whether compensation claims could be contributing to the symptoms.

➤ Post-traumatic epilepsy: head injury is the cause of 2% of epilepsy cases. Early seizures (within the first week of the injury) are more common than late onset seizures. Depressed skull fractures, intracranial haematoma, prolonged post-traumatic amnesia (> 24 hours), dural tear and early seizures increase the risk of post-traumatic epilepsy.

➤ Loss of the sense of smell (anosmia) as a result of head injury is usually permanent due to damage of the olfactory (1st) nerve.

➤ Chronic subdural haematoma: usually occurs in older people and alcoholics after a minor head injury. Patients present with headaches and drowsiness weeks after the head injuries. Brain CT is diagnostic and surgical evacuation is needed. If missed, patients develop focal neurological signs and coma. They may die as a result of increased intracranial pressure leading to coning.

➤ After a head injury patients may have behavioural and psychological problems, impairment of memory and permanent neurological deficit (hemiplegia).

CHAPTER 29

Other neurological disorders

This chapter includes a brief description of neurological disorders not included in the other chapters.

DEGENERATIVE DISC DISEASE

➤ Common in clinical practice, especially in the cervical and lumbosacral areas.
➤ Usually due to the formation of osteophytes or degeneration of interverterbral discs.
➤ Can cause nerve root lesion (radiculopathy), which leads to pain with or without sensory or motor symptoms and signs of urinary bladder impairment.
➤ A common cause of acute or chronic spinal cord compression (cervical cord) and cauda equina syndrome (spinal cord ends at L1/2 level; therefore the nerve roots from lumbar and sacral segments of the spinal cord have to travel a relatively long distance before exiting the spinal canal, forming a horse tail-like structure called the cauda equina).
➤ MRI of the spine and NCS and/or EMG are helpful in making a diagnosis.

➤ Management includes pain relief, physiotherapy and surgical measures.

FUNCTIONAL DISORDERS

➤ Functional disorders usually refers to patients with neurological symptoms but no disease. They are common in neurological practice.
➤ Many terms have been used:
  ➢ functional
  ➢ non-organic
  ➢ psychogenic
  ➢ psychosomatic
  ➢ medically unexplained
  ➢ abnormal illness behaviour
  ➢ conversion disorders
  ➢ somatisation disorders
  ➢ hysteria.
➤ Patients who *consciously* fabricate symptoms are described as:
  ➢ *Factitious* – if the purpose is to get medical care and attention
  ➢ *Munchausen* – if a patient with a factitious disorder get medical care (usually emergency departments and inpatients) in different hospitals (wanders between doctors and hospitals)
  ➢ *Malingering* – factitious disorder for material gain.
➤ The most common presentations of patient with functional disorders in neurology practice are:
  ➢ *Non-epileptic attack disorder* – *see* Chapter 18.
  ➢ *Weakness* – usually develops suddenly. There is always a degree of inconsistency (patient able to walk but can't lift the leg up off the bed).
  ➢ *Gait disorders* – patient may swing from side to side in a very unusual way. This can be mistakenly labelled as ataxic gait.
  ➢ *Tremor* – tends to be easily distractable.
  ➢ *Sensory symptoms* – impairment of sensation in exactly one-half of the body (split in half).

➤ Investigations and over-investigations with repeated scans are usually inescapable.

➤ Patients need a full explanation about the problem. Some patients find it difficult to accept that there is no physical cause for their symptoms. The way the diagnosis is explained to the patient is vital.

➤ Further referral to psychiatry, psychology or neuropsychiatry is helpful. However, it is vital that the psychiatrist, psychologist or neuropsychiatrist has an interest in functional disorders otherwise it may make things worse!

➤ Cognitive behavioural therapy may help.

➤ Physiotherapy for patients with gait disorders or weakness is useful.

➤ The earlier the diagnosis is made the better the outcome.

HUNTINGTON'S DISEASE

➤ An autosomal dominant neurodegenerative disorder.

➤ HD is due to the expanded trinucleotide cytosine-adenine-guanine repeat on chromosome 4. Diagnostic genetic test for the trinucleotide repeat is widely available.

➤ HD presents with the following:
  ➣ chorea (involuntary, irregular, fidgety and random movements)
  ➣ dementia
  ➣ psychiatric problems.

➤ There is no specific treatment. Genetic counselling can be offered to the family members.

MYOTONIC DYSTROPHY

➤ An autosomal dominant disorder.

➤ Myotonic dystrophy is due to the expanded trinucleotide repeat and a diagnostic genetic test is widely available.

➤ Patients usually have:
  ➣ Characteristic facial appearance (frontal baldness, ptosis, wasting of masseter and temporalis muscles, bilateral facial weakness).

➤ Myotonia – to demonstrate, ask the patient to make a tight fist and release it; there will be a delay in relaxing the hand. By striking the thenar eminence with a tendon hammer, percussion myotonia can be seen; it will take a long time for the dimple to return to normal.
➤ Cataract.
➤ Cardiac conduction defects.
➤ Diabetes.
➤ Testicular atrophy.
➤ Impairment of intellectual function.
➤ EMG will show evidence of myotonia.
➤ There is no specific treatment. Genetic counselling can be offered to the family members. Cardiac monitoring with regular ECG. Regular checking of blood sugar.

PLEXOPATHY

➤ Plexopathy is a disorder of the brachial or lumbosacral plexus. Brachial plexopathy is more common than lumbosacral plexopathy.
➤ Usually causes pain, weakness and sensory symptoms and signs.
➤ The causes of plexopathy include the following:
  ➤ possible viral infection or immunisation (brachial neuritis)
  ➤ neoplastic infiltration
  ➤ radiation
  ➤ trauma and injuries due to invasive medical procedures.
➤ MRI of plexus and NCS and/or EMG are helpful in making the diagnosis.
➤ Treatment is usually supportive (pain relief and physiotherapy) and treatment of the underlying cause (malignancies) if possible.

SYRINGOMYELIA

➤ Syringomyelia is a rare neurology condition resulting from abnormal fluid collection (syrinx) within several segments of the spinal cord (myelia) usually the cervical or thoracic cord. It may extend to the medulla (syringobulbia).
➤ It is associated with Chiari's malformation (the medulla and the

lower part of the cerebellum descend below the level of foramen magnum). Trauma and tumour of the spinal cord can cause syringomyelia. Some cases are idiopathic.

➤ Patients usually present with:
  ➢ loss of pain and temperature sensation leading to burning marks in the upper limbs
  ➢ wasting, weakness and loss of reflexes in the upper limbs
  ➢ spastic legs.
➤ MRI of the spine is diagnostic.
➤ Surgical treatment should be considered.

SUBACUTE COMBINED DEGENERATION OF THE SPINAL CORD

➤ Subacute combined degeneration of the spinal cord is due to vitamin B_{12} deficiency, leading to dysfunction of the dorsal columns (impairment of vibration and position sense) and corticospinal tracts (causing motor weakness).
➤ Patients present with balance problems and weak legs. Neurological examination shows sensory ataxia, spastic legs with absent ankle reflexes and upgoing plantars.
➤ Patients should be treated with vitamin B_{12} injections.

MUSCLE DISEASES

➤ Muscle diseases are relatively rare in clinical practice.
➤ Patients usually show sign of proximal myopathy (weakness around the hip and shoulder girdles). Patient has difficulty standing from the sitting position. Muscle diseases can involve the respiratory and cardiac muscles.
➤ Patients can have a waddling gait (*see* p. 26).
➤ The following are causes of muscle diseases:
  ➢ Polymyositis or dermatomyositis – they occur in isolation or are associated with other autoimmune diseases. Dermatomyositis is associated with skin changes such as heliotrope rash and photosensitive rash. Also, dermatomyositis is associated with malignancy.
  ➢ Inclusion body myositis, which is the most common form

of myopathy after the age of 50. Involvement of finger flexors, foot extensors and quadriceps are early pointers to the diagnosis.

➤ Endocrine causes – Cushing's syndrome and thyrotoxicosis.

➤ Drug-induced myopathies – steroids, amiodarone, lithium and statins.

➤ Genetic myopathies – includes muscular dystrophies such as Duchenne and Becker types of muscular dystrophy and limb girdle dystrophy.

➤ Metabolic myopathies such as mitochondrial disorders, acid maltase deficiency and myophosphorylase deficiency.

➤ Alcoholism.

➤ Osteomalacia.

➤ The following investigations are usually needed:

➤ blood tests, such as thyroid function test

➤ muscle enzymes

➤ EMG

➤ muscle biopsy

➤ genetic testing.

➤ Depending on the type of muscle disease, some disorders are not treatable and only supportive measures are available. Other diseases, such as polymyositis and dermatomyositis, are treatable usually by corticosteroids and other immunosuppressive agents such as azathioprine and methotrexate.

CHARCOT–MARIE–TOOTH DISEASE

➤ CMT, or hereditary motor and sensory neuropathy, is mainly an autosomal dominant disease causing predominantly motor peripheral neuropathy.

➤ Patients present with bilateral distal wasting and weakness of ankle dorsiflexion (bilateral foot drop), pes cavus and absent ankle and knee jerks. There may be wasting of the small muscles of the hand and absent upper limb reflexes.

➤ The degree of disability is usually minimal, in spite of the marked neurological signs.

➤ Patient may have a high steppage gait (*see* p. 26).

➤ CMT can cause both demyelinating and axonal neuropathy.
➤ NCS and/or EMG and genetic testing, duplication of the gene PMP22 (peripheral myelin protein 22) help in making the diagnosis.
➤ Patients need supportive measures such as physiotherapy, splints and genetic counselling.

NARCOLEPSY

➤ Patients with narcolepsy present with excessive daytime sleepiness (an irresistible urge to sleep).
➤ Narcolepsy is usually associated with:
  ➤ *Cataplexy* – sudden loss of muscle tone (without losing consciousness) leading to falls. This is provoked by laughter or other emotional stimulus.
  ➤ *Sleep paralysis* – patient is fully awake but cannot move. It is a frightening experience.
  ➤ *Hypnagogic hallucinations* – another frightening experience. Usually visual hallucinations occur as the patient is drifting off to sleep.
➤ CNS stimulants such as modafinil and dexamphetamine are used to treat narcolepsy, while cataplexy, sleep paralysis and hypnagogic hallucinations respond to tricyclic antidepressants and selective serotonin reuptake inhibitors.

Index